THE BEST DOCTORS
IN THE U.S.

*A Guide to the Finest Specialists,
Hospitals, and Health Centers*

THE BEST DOCTORS IN THE U.S.

A Guide to the Finest Specialists, Hospitals, and Health Centers

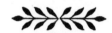

JOHN PEKKANEN

Seaview Books

NEW YORK

FIRST EDITION

Trade distribution by Simon and Schuster
A Division of Gulf + Western Corporation
New York, New York 10020

Designed by Tere LoPrete

Library of Congress Cataloging in Publication Data

Pekkanen, John, 1939–
  The best doctors in the U.S.

  1. Physicians—United States—Directories.
2. Physicians—United States—Rating of. 3. Medicine—
Specialties and specialists—United States—Directories.
4. Hospitals—United States—Directories. 5. Medical
centers—United States—Directories. I. Title.
R712.A1P44   610'.25'73   79–15983
ISBN 0–87223–533–5 (Seaview Books trade edition)
ISBN 0–87223–580–7 (Wideview Books paperback edition)

Contents

For physicians of excellence everywhere

Contents

Acknowledgments

If I were to acknowledge all of the individuals who are responsible for this book, there would be nearly 550 names; these would be the physicians who took the time to assist me in this project. Because all of them spoke to me in confidence, I cannot reveal their names. However, I especially want to thank those who gave me large amounts of their time and who were especially encouraging to me in this endeavor. I cannot repay their patience, advice, and help, but they should know that I am in their debt and that without their help this project would not have been possible.

I owe a special thanks to four people at *Town & Country*, where this project was initiated and where an earlier and much abbreviated form of it first appeared. Ms. Lorraine Dusky, then an editor at the magazine, first talked with me about this project, and those conversations led to articles and eventually to this book. Ms. Barbara King worked on the project in its latter stages and offered thoughtful and constructive advice. Ms. Missy Becker did a mammoth amount of checking and rechecking of my facts and interpretations and caught many uncorrected errors. Finally, Frank Zachary, the editor-in-chief at *Town & Country*, first offered me the opportunity to do this project and then the encouragement to keep at it when it appeared impossibly difficult. His enthusiasm was contagious and his compassion and intelligence inspiring. All four of these individuals are professionals in every good sense of that word, and I shall not forget their enormous contributions to this project.

My editor on this book, Charles Sopkin, was equally encouraging and thoughtful through the many stages of assembling the information for this project. I owe him a debt for that alone, and also for his acute awareness of the medical profession and for the guidance and advice he gave me.

Ms. Jane Silver helped me on some research aspects of this project, and her assistance was greatly valued. Ms. Barbara Crandall typed portions of this book and correctly interpreted many of my scribblings.

Finally, I wish publicly to thank my wife, Lynn, for her constant support through all phases of this project. Besides her substantive contributions to this project, she kept our whole family on an even keel through the most difficult phases of this project.

I want to add one final note. This book has not received the direct or indirect support of anyone other than my publisher. I did not seek support from any governmental, philanthropic, or medical organization, nor would I have accepted any if it had been offered. This book was and is an independent enterprise undertaken solely to promote greater public awareness of how to get the best medical treatment.

Introduction

The reason this book was written can be stated very simply: There is an enormous variation in the quality of medical care in this country and that variation can mean the difference between life and death. The specific purpose of this book is to guide you to the best in medical care.

The Subcommittee on Oversight and Investigations of the House of Representatives reported in its 1978 report on surgical performance: "An individual may have *twice* the chance of dying from an operation simply by having the procedure performed at one hospital rather than another. The Subcommittee finds that the information now being made available to the public concerning quality of care is not adequate."

The quality of medical care varies not only from one hospital to the next, but considerably within the same hospital, depending on your doctor. A doctor who is known as an exacting physician who puts his patient's welfare before anything else will get maximum efficiency from the hospital staff—the residents, nurses, and all the other health care professionals. However, if he is not exacting, he will not inspire the staff to be efficient. One doctor put it this way: "There are two levels of care in the same hospital. The top level goes to those patients who have doctors that demand it. The second level of care goes to those patients whose doctors are known to the hospital staff to be lazy or sloppy."

Although it is disturbing that there is a considerable amount of mediocre—or worse—medical care in the country, it is encouraging to know that there are a significant number of doctors who are gifted and dedicated in their pursuit of the best medical care for their patients.

It is important that laymen learn to recognize a good doctor when they see one, a task that is often very difficult. In a classic study made fifteen years ago under the direction of Doctors Ray E. Trussell and M. A. Morehead—a study still valid today—a careful survey of surgical and medical care of hundreds of patients in 100 hospitals in the New York City area found that 43 percent of the care was less than good and 23 percent was poor. Yet, the study found, the patients were "overwhelmingly" satisfied with their care. Many laymen are caught up in or confused by the mystique of medicine. They don't understand the process or the language. And all too often malpractice suits are brought for problems of communication between patient and doctor, rather than for actual malpractice. Considerable malpractice and malfeasance go unreported or unnoticed, particularly in the area of unnecessary surgery. Some estimates report that more than *two million* unnecessary surgical procedures are performed each year.

Many laymen also tend to believe there is more science to medicine than there actually is. In fact, there is as much art as science to it. Diagnosis and treatment are not well-formulated, reflective responses by doctors. Diagnosis of the same symptoms can differ dramatically, as can treatment for the same disease. These differences can and do mean a good result or a bad one and, in the most extreme cases, the difference between life and death.

This book was designed and written to put vital medical information into your hands—the patient's hands—that will enable you to make sounder medical decisions for yourself and your family.

The book does this in two ways: First, it describes precisely what doctors themselves regard as the most important qualifications for a doctor to possess; second, it offers a specific name-by-name guide to many of the best specialists, hospitals, clinics, and special centers in this country and Canada. The specialists who are included in this book are the doctors' doctors. These are the specialized physicians whom other doctors regard as outstanding in their field and to whom they would turn if they or their family were struck with serious illness. This is information that has long been used by the doctors themselves when they are faced with personal medical crises. Now this book enables you to use it to get better health care for you and your family.

The Making of This Book

The research for this book extended over a period of a year and a half, but the effort was not full-time for all eighteen months. It began in 1977 with research into an article for *Town & Country* magazine, which resulted in a two-part section on the best medical service. The article named several, but by no means all, medical specialties and outstanding individuals in them. The article was based on confidential interviews with more than eighty medical specialists around the country. They were asked to name the doctors in their own specialties they considered outstanding; these would be the doctors they would consult if they had a medical problem covered by their own specialty.

With the decision to begin this book, I mailed confidential questionnaires to the more than 500 physicians who appeared in the original article. (About 2,500 names appear in this book.) I mailed them the questionnaires against the advice of several physician friends of mine who warned that doctors would not take the time to answer them and I was wasting time and money. I mailed them nonetheless and asked, in my covering letter, this question: "If you or a member of your family were ill with a problem in your own specialty, who would you go to for treatment?" Although the questionnaire also asked for recommendations in other specialties, experience had taught me that physicians are most knowledgeable about doctors within their own specialties and subspecialties. I, of course, guaranteed absolute confidentiality and stated, and continue to state, that the name of no one who communicated with me would be divulged without his or her consent. For this reason, none of the quotes in this book are attributed.

I expected a 10 percent return and hoped for a 20 percent return. In fact, I received a total of 310 completed questionnaires, or a total return rate of just over 60 percent. The vast majority of the returns were very helpful. Many encouraged the project, saying it was an important contribution to quality control in medical care. A few of the returns questioned the idea, but only two flatly opposed it. Also, only two doctors said they did not wish their names to be included. One said he had retired, the other was editing a medical journal and was no longer seeing patients.

One who opposed the idea suggested it was not possible to find the names of all the outstanding physicians in the country with such a limited sample. He argued that I would have to interview hundreds of individuals in each specialty alone. On the first point I am in agreement. There is no possible way for this book or any other similar enterprise to properly evaluate and list the names of all the outstanding physicians in this country. Even if you grant that only the top 10 percent of the physicians in the country are truly superior, this would mean there are at least 30,000 first-rate doctors in the country. As noted, this book includes about 2,500 names.

On the second point I disagree, however. I did multiple interviewing in every specialty to find the outstanding individuals included in this book. I cross-checked each name against several doctors in each specialty. In many instances, those checks and rechecks *reduced* the number of doctors listed rather than increased it. Thus, it is my experience that a substantially larger sample may not produce a substantially larger number of truly outstanding doctors for these lists.

The wealth of information I received on the returned questionnaires was collected, and doctors suggested which specialties I should include, and some outstanding people in them. They suggested various special centers where unusual types of medical care are given. In some cases, the doctors added no new names for me but indicated by filling in an optional part of the questionnaire that they would talk candidly with me in a personal interview or by telephone. However, the vast majority of the returned questionnaires included new names. One questionnaire came back with ninety-one names of suggested physicians. This was far and away the record. Second place was forty-six names. My suspicion, which was usually correct, was that no one doctor could vouch for so many names and remain certain of their quality.

My next step was to evaluate the names, and to do this I selected key individuals in each of the specialties. How did I decide they were key people? In most cases, they were individuals cited by a number of their peers as truly outstanding, doctors that other doctors looked up to. I had no preconception as to how long each list should be or where the individuals should come from. In other words, I was not reaching to find the best doctor in any one area. Rather, I was seeking truly outstanding doctors, and if they did not spread geographically, then so be it. However, because there are outstanding medical schools and facilities in most parts of the country, doctors in all parts of the country showed up in many different specialties.

The evaluation of the lists and individuals on it took more than six full months and 185 additional interviews. Only one doctor I contacted by phone refused to comment. Some of the interviews were relatively brief, others lasted for hours. Many were personal visits, most were by telephone. Thus, including the eighty originally interviewed for the magazine article and the 185 interviewed specifically for the book, and the 310 questionnaires which were returned, and accounting for the fact that some doctors overlap in all these areas, I was in direct communication with a total of 545 doctors in preparing this book. They came from all parts of the country and from all levels of medicine. Some were mostly in private practice with a loose medical school affiliation, some were assistant or associate or full professors, others were chairmen of medical departments at the country's finest medical schools. Some were government employees of the National Institutes of Health. In all, more than eighty medical institutions were represented.

There was nothing magical about the number of doctors I interviewed. It was just that 545 was the number that I reached when I felt sufficiently confident that all of the specialties were graced with outstanding specialists. For each specialty, specialists were interviewed in depth to find and confirm and reconfirm who the outstanding people are.

Besides seeking outstanding quality, I was also seeking "good doctors." That is, I asked doctors to evaluate other doctors on the basis of their rapport with and sympathy for people. In one instance, I brought up the name of a doctor to another doctor, who commented: "There is no question that he is bright and knowledgeable, but he is a beast with people. He is unbelievably rude and for that reason I'd never go to him." In cases such as this, when it was clear that the doctor in question was inept at dealing with people to the point that even doctors who respected his skill would not see him, the name was excluded.

How did the doctors I spoke with judge superiority? In all cases, individuals are named who have had extensive contact over a number of years with other doctors. These dealings include mutual patient referrals, meeting with them at the gatherings of the various medical societies, and reading their medical writings. "When you read what another doctor has written," one physician said, "you really see how his mind works. You can tell very quickly if he is at the top of his field."

Doctors also serve as visiting professors at other medical schools and learn intimately how other doctors relate to their patients and to colleagues. Surgeons watch other surgeons in other cities perform surgery, and they also watch them operate via films shown at medical meetings. Also, in many, many cases, doctors have trained other doctors. As one doctor said, "When you train a man you learn a tremendous amount about him, his judgment, his skills, how he sizes up a situation."

In many instances doctors would mention an individual and tell me at the same time that they personally did not like him but, they would add, "He is an outstanding doctor." On the other hand, physicians would not want to include some physicians even though they were close personal friends. "He just isn't top rank," would be a frequent comment. It became clear from my interviewing that doctors do in fact have very detailed and intimate knowledge of their colleagues in their own medical specialties.

In a very real sense, the upper level of the medical profession operates as a small, elite national society. It knows no regional bounds. When I talked to a doctor in California, he was just as likely to name an outstanding individual in New York as was someone living in his own city.

However, while many physicians have a reputation, which may or may not be deserved, it was clear in every interview that physicians know the doctors they recommend not only by reputation but well enough so that they would go to them for their own medical problems. I frequently asked surgeons, "If you were lying on the operating table and looked up and saw (doctor's name), would you feel at ease?" There would sometimes be a pause, but when the answer came, I knew it was well considered.

I also placed a special emphasis on finding out about a doctor's local reputation, which can sometimes be far different from his national reputation. In some cases this proved to be decisive, but in most cases those doctors who are most respected nationally are also well respected at home. "Sometimes a big reputation can go to a doctor's head," one doctor said. "He gets pretty full of himself and forgets his job back home is to take care of sick people."

Many excellent physicians were overlooked because they do not publish or attend the meetings of the various medical societies and thus do not come to the attention of their peers. Also, many of the country's most brilliant doctors are researchers and do not see patients. The vast majority of doctors on this list are researchers-clinicians, that is, they do both research and patient care. Still others were not included because they have retired, and others, although considered outstanding, are now involved in so much administrative work that they have little, if any, time for patients.

Reputations are most quickly and visibly established through research because it is published in the medical journals and comes to the attention of the physicians in that field. Thus, individuals who do research and publish their findings become more widely known than their colleagues who do not do research. Although research skills do not translate into clinical skills (an individual who may know everything about a disease may still not be able to diagnose or treat it well), they are an indication that the physician not only is "keeping up" but is at the cutting edge of his profession. It is probably the single most important factor which places some doctors over others.

However, while reputation was important, it was more important to determine how the reputation was established. If it was established by research, specialists were well equipped to decide whether the research was in fact a significant contribution to their field or whether it was, as one doctor called it, "a rearrangement of other people's data."

In some cases, a reputation goes with the title, particularly when that title is a prestigious one from a prestigious university. However, these can be very misleading. One story well known in medical circles involves a chaired professorship at Harvard University. Several years ago the chair was held by one of the most widely respected men in his specialty. He was known for his vast knowledge of his field as well as his clinical skill. When he retired, his chair was given to another man. Thus, by elevation to this chair, that man assumed a major reputation in his field. But, as one doctor who recounted this incident recalled: "This doctor turned out to have no clinical skill whatever, and almost no teaching skills. It took some time for the message to go around the world, but he soon stopped being consulted and so did his entire department. When he left the department, partly by invitation, it was a shambles." The point of the story is a simple one. There can be an enormous gap between reputation and quality. Every effort was made in the research into this book to make that differentiation and to list only those with well-earned reputations and whose quality was respected.

These qualifications and considerations went into selecting those outstanding individuals listed here. I devised no rigid formulas to judge the doctors to include or not to include. Such formulas would have been useless because the circumstances changed from case to case. It is sufficient to say that every name in this book was weighed carefully by several specialists in each field. Always the question asked of doctors was: Would you have him as your doctor? And, finally, I asked myself the question: Knowing what I know, would I use him as my doctor? When those questions could be answered affirmatively, the doctor was included.

Perhaps what has most surprised individuals who have known about this project is the fact that doctors have spoken to me so willingly. Doctors have the reputation of never speaking bluntly of their colleagues. From previous experience in medical writing, I knew that this was not true. Still, I had some reservations as to how open doctors would be in commenting specifically on their colleagues—both positively and negatively. That lingering doubt was forever dispelled during one interview very early in this project. I called a well-known and well-respected specialist whom I did not know and who did not know me. I discussed the project with him and gave him the names of some other individuals in his specialty. He approved of them all except one, of whom he said: "I wouldn't take my dog to that quack." His remarks, although blunter than most, were echoed by scores of physicians I spoke with. They spoke openly about their profession and their colleagues. I asked several of them why they were being this frank, and this is basically what they told me: They regard the medical profession as troubled. It is beset by staggering costs, by a troublesome amount of unprofessionalism in its ranks, and by an anti-doctor climate reflected in part by the rising number of malpractice suits.

These doctors said they were being this candid and helpful because they honestly felt that this project would serve to upgrade their profession and assist the public in dealing with doctors. "I think," one doctor said, "the public has a full right to know who we think are the best in our profession. We certainly know who the best doctors are. I think you'll find that physicians who are loath to say anything publicly against another doctor fear reprisals and simply don't want to get embroiled in a name-calling contest. But in private we express very strong opinions about who is good and who isn't. Those opinions are openly shared among us."

Guaranteed confidentiality, the more than 500 doctors I communicated with were extremely candid and open. Some were extraordinarily helpful, giving me hours of their time and enormous amounts of good advice. In addition, I selected doctors in every specialty to read each section for accuracy, and many offered suggestions that have greatly improved this book.

What Is a Good Doctor and How Should You Choose Him or Her?

As part of my research for this book, I tried to find those qualities doctors seek in their *own* doctors. In particular, I asked doctors themselves what they considered important objective qualifications for outstanding doctors. Basically, I sought to find methods by which laymen could make better and more informed judgments of their own physicians.

The reasoning behind this is two-fold. First, although great effort has been expended to make this book as complete as possible in identifying outstanding specialists, it is by no means complete. As I have said before, there are many outstanding physicians in active practice that are not named in this book. Second, many physicians in this book are not primary care doctors. Many are surgeons who perform surgery and care for the patient pre- and postoperatively, but do not take day-to-day care of the patient. Still others do consultative work for specific medical problems and are not available for ongoing care. I should add, however, that there are a substantial number of physicians listed here who do take primary care of patients with certain medical problems.

Doctors also felt that patients should have more decision-making power over their own care. They agreed patients should be more aware of the background of their doctor and more aware of those factors that may indicate he or she is of superior (or inferior) quality. "It is really the best way to police our profession," one doctor said. "If people become better informed, doctors will have to improve or they'll have fewer patients."

To their credit, many outstanding doctors believe laymen should know more about the medical profession. They feel medicine should be demythologized and should be made more accessible. In this section, I have tried to distill the ways doctors think and the criteria they consider important in selecting doctors for themselves.

It is crucial that you be very careful in selecting any doctor for yourself. To be casual about the selection of a family doctor because you only rely on him to treat the usual run of illnesses is a mistake. It is your family doctor or general internist who is your entry point into the medical system. In case of serious illness, he refers you to a specialist or to a hospital. If he is an excellent doctor, he will likely refer you to other excellent doctors. Like other professionals, doctors travel in spheres of excellence, and a good doctor will rarely recommend a poor one. A poor doctor will more likely refer you to another poor doctor. Said one doctor: "I believe that virtually every practicing physician does indeed want the very best result from the treatment of his patients. I do not believe that he deliberately denies this opportunity to any of his patients. The major problem seems to be that the truly complicated problem constitutes only a very small fraction of the patients in his practice. I think the physician often fails to recognize a disaster which is staring him in the face until it is often too late."

The following, not listed in order of importance, are the factors doctors say you should consider when selecting a physician for yourself.

Board Certification. In the questionnaire I posed a question: "What importance do you attach to board certification for judging the competence of physicians?" Four options were listed: very significant; significant; insignificant; other (explain). The response was overwhelmingly in support of board certification as an important factor in choosing a doctor. Of those 310 who responded to the questionnaire, 294 (95 percent) said they considered board certification to be either significant or very significant. In commenting on board certification, one doctor said: "It is significant only to assure *minimum* competence." Another said: "It is most significant when a patient is unfamiliar with doctors in his geographical area. There are few good specialists who are not board certified." Another noted: "It establishes the doctor has been exposed to what his peers regard as suitable training. More importantly, it indicates that he is aware of the public and that the requirements of medical care demand some sort of tangible measurement of training, experience, and reliability and that he is willing to live within an established system even though it has many flaws." Finally, one physician noted: "If a physician has it (board certification), I am not impressed. If he doesn't have it, I consider it to be a very serious mark against him."

What precisely is board certification? In a general sense, board certification is a process by which the medical profession has established basic standards of knowledge and skill for its physicians. It is a *minimum* standard. In essence, to be board certified, a physician must have graduated from medical school, completed his residency and two or three years of supervised specialty training at an approved medical institution.

If the doctor is attempting to be board certified in surgery, he must keep a detailed log of the surgery he performed, the indications for it, the complications that arose, and the results. If he is seeking board certification in internal medicine, he must also complete the approved postgraduate training in that specialty. In addition, a critique of his or her performance must be made by the physician supervising the postgraduate fellowship program. At this point, the applicant becomes "board eligible" and can take the board examination. It is a full-day test, and in every specialty it is geared toward clinical care. Each specialty devises its own tests. Many of the tests are written so an applicant is given a medical problem and is given a choice as to what to do. Through a series of follow-up questions, he is asked to analyze this and other medical situations fully. In addition to the written questions, there is an oral examination. The oral examiners are selected on the basis of their acknowledged experience and expertise in each of the specialty areas. One board examiner spoke of the experience: "Usually, within a very short time, I can tell who the graduates of the best medical schools and best residency programs are. You can see very quickly that they are the most assured, the most knowledgeable, the most experienced. Although we looked for specific detailed knowledge on the part of the applicant, we also looked for character. I am most impressed by applicants who are honest, who will tell you they don't know the answer to a question rather than trying to fake their way through it. I think this is an important quality in a doctor and it is something we look for in our board examinations."

Of all the applicants who take the boards, about two-thirds to three-quarters of them pass. (Some are marked on a curve.) Those who do not pass remain eligible for two more board examinations. If they fail them, it is very difficult for them to secure a fourth examination. The vast majority of physicians who fail three times never become board certified.

What are the flaws of board certification? The most obvious major flaw is that passing a test is not necessarily a good indication that a physician will make a superior patient care physician. It is, as most all doctors attest, only a minimum guarantee. It is a minimum guarantee especially for those who pass the boards by a minimum score. Board certification is only a guarantee that the physician has passed through an approved training program, that his or her medical performance has been scrutinized by critical eyes, and that he or she has demonstrated at least a theoretical grasp of medicine in his or her particular specialty.

Failing the boards also does not in any way prevent a physician from practicing medicine—any kind of medicine that he chooses. However, board certification has taken on enormous significance at university-affiliated medical centers. In these centers, a physician who is not board certified and is not board eligible (meaning he has failed the exam three times) has virtually no chance of practicing medicine. There is no question that board certification is an imperfect tool by which to measure doctors. But it remains an important guide to a physician's training, and, at the very least, his minimum understanding of that training. At present there is no requirement for recertification. However, there is movement to establish recertification after five, seven, or perhaps ten years. However, as expected, many physicians are resisting this.

How can you find out if a doctor is board certified? One way is to ask him or her, but most people are too embarrassed to be that direct. Another way is to call your local medical society. And yet another way is to look him or her up in the *Directory of Medical Specialists*. This is a large, two-volume book which includes the name of *every* physician in this country and abroad who has passed his or her U.S. specialty boards. The directory is available at all medical libraries and is also available at many public libraries. Physicians are listed by specialty, country, state, and city, and one of the volumes has a complete alphabetical index of all the names and the pages where their professional biographies appear.

One note of caution: Many entries in the book are out-of-date. Doctors who have very recently passed their boards may not be included even in the most recent editions of the directory. This fact notwithstanding, the directory is a valuable source of information on physicians. It provides substantial objective information on a doctor's training. Besides his specialty board certification, it also indicates if he has passed his subspecialty boards. Subspecialty boards are significant in internal medicine because they subdivide the different specialties within internal medicine into cardiology, gastroenterology, endocrinology, and others. Although many physicians do not consider the subspecialty boards as crucial as the specialty boards, the directory nonetheless will show if in fact a doctor who says he is a cardiologist has passed his subspecialty board in cardiology.

A second note of caution: Although board certification is a very important consideration in choosing a doctor, it is also important to take into account the age of the doctor when you consider it. Because many of the specialty boards are relatively new—some subspecialty boards were established only in the 1970s—many older doctors have not taken them. In some cases, older doctors are given "grandfather" certificates on the basis of their medical experience, but this is not true with all the boards. Thus, age is an important consideration. Also, some doctors who have failed their boards twice may continue to say they are "board eligible" when they may have no intention of trying to pass their boards again. If a doctor is beyond his early forties and continues to maintain that he is board eligible, you can rightly be wary of him. As one doctor so bluntly said, "If you are in a doctor's office and he is under the age of fifty and he isn't board certified, walk out of his office."

Residency Training. Another critical aspect of a physician's training is his residency. This is the period after graduation from medical school in which he or she spends three years in working and training as a doctor at a hospital. During residency training, physicians go on different services at different periods of time in order to subject themselves to all areas of medical care. They may be on cardiology for three months and then on general surgery.

Where a physician does his residency training is very critical to his development as a doctor, and the best hospitals in which to do residency training are university-affiliated hospitals. One physician said: "It is my opinion that residency training at the worst university-affiliated hospital is better than residency training at the best nonuniversity-affiliated hospital." In the course of researching this book, I asked a number of physicians if they agreed with this statement. All but one did. The lone dissenter said he agreed with it in almost all cases, but he believed there were a few selected private hospitals where residency programs were excellent.

Why are university-affiliated residency programs superior? Largely because university hospitals are fishbowls in which everything a doctor does is watched and criticized by his peers. It is this critical, questioning environment and the fact that individuals who staff university hospitals are in the business of teaching and training doctors that makes these programs superior. At most private hospitals the medical staff is not set up to do this.

If you wish to find out where a doctor has done his residency it will be listed in the *Directory of Medical Specialists* if he is already board certified. However, the fact that he is board certified carries greater weight than where he did his residency. However, if he is board eligible or is not yet listed in the directory, you can ask his office at which hospitals he did his residency. You can then check those hospitals in the *Association of American Medical Colleges (AAMC) Directory of American Medical Education.* Under each medical school is listed the hospitals that are affiliated with it.

Medical School. Virtually every physician interviewed on this subject said he attached little significance to the medical school a physician attended, as long as it was a U.S. medical school. U.S. and Canadian medical schools, and those of Great Britain, are considered the best in the world. Many doctors expressed serious reservations about the quality of other foreign medical schools in which 6,000 U.S. citizens are now enrolled.

In a special article in the *New England Journal of Medicine* of October 19, 1978, a comparison was made of standardized test scores achieved by U.S. citizens who graduated from foreign medical schools versus those of graduates of U.S. medical schools. The percentage of U.S. and Canadian medical school graduates who passed the tests in 1975 and 1976, respectively, was 79 percent and 81 percent. The percentage of U.S. citizens educated in foreign medical schools who passed the tests in the same two years was 18 and 16 percent, respectively. Four times as many U.S. educated medical students passed the same tests as foreign educated U.S. citizens.

Although all tests are limited in what they display of a person's knowledge, intelligence, and judgment, these test results do comport with the opinion of many physicians that foreign medical schools are generally inferior to U.S., Canadian, and English medical schools. However, there are exceptions to any rule, and many foreign trained doctors, both U.S. citizens and foreign citizens, have become outstanding.

University Affiliation. Every physician interviewed on this subject said he would consider a university affiliation significant in choosing any doctor for himself. "A university affiliation indicates an interest in continuing education, an interest in seeing what the latest developments are. I think it is vital," said one doctor who spoke for many. There is no question that my sample was biased because I interviewed so many physicians in academic medicine. However, they made the repeated point that a university affiliation usually indicates a physician intends to practice medicine at a reasonably high level. There are obviously exceptions to this rule. Some university-affiliated physicians do not practice good medicine, and some physicians with a purely private practice are superior clinical care doctors. However, a doctor who teaches is virtually forced to keep up, and that benefits the patient.

Medical Society Membership. Some surgeons regard membership in the American College of Surgeons as important. "You are nominated and elected into the American College of Surgeons," one doctor said. "You have to meet certain criteria in the eyes of your peers in order to be accepted, and not everyone is. I would want any surgeon operating on me to be a member."

There are societies for every medical specialty and for a vast number of the subspecialties. However, most of these societies accept for membership any and all certified applicants who apply. They are, therefore, not a good guide to excellence.

In many ways, selecting a doctor is an attempt at bettering your odds. There is no such thing as a sure thing. Even the best of doctors have off-days. Nevertheless, you should approach the selection of a doctor in a careful, calculated way. And by picking one who has a university affiliation, even a loose one, you are improving your odds. All too often our selection of a doctor is based on the word of a friend or neighbor. It is well to ask for opinions, but it is equally important to do your own independent checking to see if he or she measures up to the basic standards doctors themselves consider so vital to good medicine. These are the objective criteria physicians judge other physicians by. They are not guarantees, rather they are useful guides. If you are seeking a physician and know nothing about him other than that he fulfills the criteria just outlined, you are greatly improving your chances of securing a good doctor.

Beyond these objective guides, there are a number of subjective ones that physicians say are very important when they decide whether or not a physician is of outstanding quality.

Does he take time with you? Perhaps surprisingly, virtually every physician interviewed on this subject said he felt a very important sign of a good physician, no matter how exalted, is that he will take ample time with each patient. "A physician must realize he is not just there to examine people and see what's wrong with them," one eminent doctor said, "but he is also there to reassure them. This takes time and patience. If a doctor rushes you or makes you feel you are taking up his valuable time, I would personally never see him again. I recall vividly one time when I was particularly harried and I was examining a patient hurriedly. To his everlasting credit, this patient spoke up. He told me right to my face that I wasn't listening to him and I wasn't giving him enough attention. I was embarrassed and I told him he was right and I apologized to him. But I'll tell you, I never made the same mistake again. Every patient, no matter how trivial you think the problem is, deserves all of your attention and all the time that is necessary." If you think your doctor isn't taking enough time with you, tell him. If he still doesn't, drop him.

Many doctors report that there are courses now being offered to doctors on how to move a vast number of patients through their office every day. These courses—for doctors in private practice—are expressly designed to minimize time and maximize profits.

What does your doctor do if you mention you want a second opinion? This is often an embarrassing situation for a patient. You have been told by a doctor that you have (or don't have) a certain problem. Perhaps you are uneasy with his diagnosis or prognosis. You want a second opinion and you ask him for his recommendations of other doctors. His reaction to this is important. *Every* physician interviewed on this subject agreed: If your doctor balks in any way when you say you want a second opinion, you should at the very least seriously reconsider keeping him as your doctor. One physician put it bluntly: "If a doctor told me I didn't need a second opinion or he took umbrage in any way to my request for one, I simply wouldn't see him again. Any doctor who is so insecure as to not trust his diagnosis is not a doctor you want for yourself. I have had a number of patients ask me for a second opinion and I gladly give them the names of several—not just one—outstanding physicians I know. If I'm wrong in my diagnosis, I'll at least learn something."

You may, of course, encounter some very real obstacles. Some doctors are reluctant to make referrals because they fear they will lose the patient and a source of income. This problem has diminished in recent years—and only a minority of doctors would strongly resist referral to a specialist. In fact the refusal of a legitimate request for a referral is in violation of the American Medical Association's Principles of Medical Ethics, which states: "A physician should seek consultation upon request; in doubtful or difficult cases; or whenever it appears that the quality of medical care may be enhanced thereby." A doctor can be reported to your medical society for refusing your referral to a specialist. You may wish to point this out to him. However, if you can't get a referral, here is what one consultant who sees patients only on a referral basis suggested:

1. The first option is to go to another primary doctor and ask him to make the referral.

2. If you don't wish to do this, put your request for a consultation in writing and mail it to the consultant you have selected.

3. Send a letter to your primary care doctor telling him or her what you have done and requesting that your medical records be forwarded to the consultant of your choice. There is considerable variability from state to state regarding your right to your own medical records, but written requests are often honored.

You should make a copy of all your written requests for your files. If a hospital denies you your records, you may appeal to a grievance board. If a private doctor denies you your records and it is not against the law in that state, you may recover them through a civil suit. There is a specific guide for this purpose researched and published by Ralph Nader's Health Research Group. It details the various state laws and specific ways in which consumers can obtain their medical records. (It is called: *Getting Yours: A Consumer's Guide to Obtaining Your Medical Records*. The cost is $2.00. It is available by writing to the Health Research Group, 2000 P Street, NW, Washington, DC 20036.)

In most cases, the consultant will see you if your effort is sincere and it is obvious that you are having difficulty getting a referral. Many physicians listed in this book also accept self-referrals.

Does he admit when he is stumped? Doctors were insistent that a truly superior doctor will always admit when he is stumped by a medical problem. "None of us knows all the answers," one said, "but some doctors refuse to admit that, and they persist with a treatment even though they are not really certain of the diagnosis and they realize the treatment is not working well. I think part of the problem is with doctors and part is with patients who look up to doctors as high priests who can't make mistakes. They must realize we can and often do."

In a number of cases doctors were asked what they considered the most important single quality for a doctor, and many of them selected this as the most important prerequisite. "Out of this quality flows everything," said one doctor. "If a doctor has the good sense to realize he doesn't know the answer and that his patient needs one, you are more than likely in very good medical hands. On the other hand, you also want someone with enough good sense and experience to know when to let well enough alone and to explain to the patient that there is nothing they need to see a specialist about. If they insist, however, all competent doctors will refer them."

Does your doctor communicate with you? Doctors have a language of their own and it is inaccessible to the average layman. If your doctor talks to you in this language and you don't understand him, many doctors regard this as a bad sign. "A doctor's ability to communicate with a patient includes his ability to listen to a patient," one doctor said. "A physician must remember that his purpose is to make the patient feel better. This is possible even in an incurable disease. I think I would sum it up by saying if you can't understand a physician don't go and see him."

Doctors also stressed that the ability to communicate extended beyond merely explaining in lay terms a patient's diagnosis. "The doctor must explain in detail what the options are in your case and he should explain to you the risks and the benefits of different courses," one doctor said. "I also think," this doctor continued, "that when a doctor makes a recommendation he should make one that he would follow for himself or his family. I think every patient has a right to ask that very question of a doctor: If you had my problem, would you do yourself what you are recommending I do? Any doctor worth his salt will give you an honest answer."

Interest in the Whole Patient. A number of doctors believe that a quality they would demand of their own doctor is an interest in the social and family stresses caused by illness. They were critical of doctors who focus entirely on the disease and ignore the fact that the illness is extraordinarily difficult for the patient and for his family. It may be called bedside manner, or plain human sensitivity, but doctors want and need this quality as laymen do.

It is important to keep these qualities in mind. Every doctor needs them, despite his title or eminence. One doctor even regarded these qualities as more important for specialists. He reasoned: "In more specialized medicine you have a tendency to see the more serious cases and by the time people get to see you they have been examined and are obviously worried and perplexed by their problem. I think we as specialists probably need more compassion than the general practice doctor, although it is often the other way around."

Peer Reputation. These criteria and qualities are what doctors considered the most important factors. However, most important is peer reputation. It is what this book is based on. It is more important than any single criterion.

You can only determine peer reputation by asking doctors specifically about another doctor. The basic question to ask is the same one

I have asked: If you were ill, who would you want to attend you? If one doctor recommends another for a specific problem, ask the recommending doctor if he knows of this doctor's experience in that area. If he is vague or doesn't have specific answers to your question, you may well ask on what basis he is recommending him. It is your duty to ask questions and demand answers.

Another source for determining peer reputation is the local medical school. The chairman of the department in the specific medical field can be a very good source for recommendations. Also, as stated at the outset, if you are careful when you pick your primary care doctor, his referrals will likely be excellent.

How to Use This Book

This book has multiple purposes. Besides the general advice on how to pick a doctor, the various sections on the specialties also have very specific advice and recommendations made by outstanding specialists.

Also, the lists of doctors themselves can be used for both care, consulting, or as a referral base. Their purpose is to give people some specific guidance as to who many of the country's outstanding physicians are, where they are, and in what specialties and subspecialties they are particularly known. Of course, it is up to you and your doctor to choose the specialist you wish to see. Also, each patient is advised to analyze any doctor he visits to see if he or she is doing the very things the doctors agreed are signs of a superior doctor. No doctor is above these. If the doctor makes you feel uncomfortable there is no rule to say you have to stay with him.

You may also wish to discuss the fee with the doctor you choose. There is a tendency to believe that the higher a doctor's reputation rises, the higher his fee. This is not necessarily so. Many outstanding specialists charge no more for their services than do other, less skilled or less well-known doctors. One doctor said he felt no doctor should take advantage of his reputation "for his own personal financial enrichment." It is an opinion shared by many. As a patient, if you are concerned about costs you should speak frankly with your doctor about his charges before you embark on a course of treatment.

In many respects, the role of the consultant differs significantly from that of the primary care doctor. There are many individuals in this book who do only medical consultation for the more difficult problems. What should you expect from them? First and foremost, besides many of the qualifications already outlined, you should expect a decision. He should make his evaluation and his diagnosis and tell you what you should do. That is his duty. He should not equivocate unless he is stumped, and in that case he should refer you to a more specialized consultant. "As a consultant it is your duty to give that patient an answer," one prominent medical consultant said, "and then make your findings clear to his primary care doctor so the appropriate treatment can be continued."

How to See the Top Man

In many cases, the physicians listed in this book as well as other outstanding doctors are the leaders of teams. They are often not only listed for themselves, but for the general superior quality of work produced by their teams. In some cases, they may be difficult to see. If you are determined to see them personally you should be insistent. There is no substitute for your own desire to be personally attended to by the specific physician you want. Said one consultant: "I think most of us are sensitive to the fact that the patient may want us to attend them personally and most of us respond to it. It's good for our egos too. I would tell anyone who feels they must see a certain individual to let that individual know, either through their referring doctor or directly by themselves."

Appointments usually have to be made well in advance, although in serious or emergency cases many of these doctors will respond quickly. In one specific section, that of limb and digit replantation after accidental amputation, emergency telephone numbers are listed for this very purpose.

This book can serve another purpose. Doctors frequently do not refer patients out of their own institutions into another one, even if the other institution has superior people for the particular problem. Let me explain. If you are seeing a doctor and it is clear you require surgery, the doctor who refers you to a surgeon will likely refer you to one who operates at the same hospital where he has privileges. You are kept in one system. The best doctors will not do this. They put the patient's welfare first and medical politics second, and will refer you to another hospital in the same city if they think there is a better surgeon or specialist there. One doctor who does this remarked: "It causes problems sometimes. Other doctors gripe that you're letting down the hospital, but if you're truly concerned about your patient you send him where you think he'll get the best treatment. Unfortunately, few of my colleagues do this enough."

Once you have settled on an excellent doctor, he will assemble the required individuals needed for your care. In many cases, because most of the outstanding specialists are affiliated with medical schools, you will be admitted to a university hospital if your problem requires hospitalization. University hospitals may be less commodious than private hospitals, but they are superior medically, a factor that could be vital if your problem is complex or if unexpected complications arise.

In the final sense, you are the one making the decisions about yourself. This book is expressly designed to assist you in making those decisions and choices. It is designed to lead you to the best in medical care because the best medical care can truly do wondrous things to combat illness.

Finally, this book is designed to put more medical decision-making power in your—the patient's—hands. It is not for the patient to diagnose and treat his illness, but it is for him to carefully weigh his medical options and to make informed choices based on knowledge and good sense rather than on blind faith.

PART I

Adult Medical, Surgical, and Diagnostic Specialists

Diseases of the
Cardiovascular System

Cardiologists

Coronary heart disease is epidemic in this country, and over the past several years there have been many new cardiologists trained to handle the very heavy caseload presented by the American public.

Cardiologists should perform two vital functions for patients.

1. They should diagnose the patient and accord him treatment appropriate to his condition.

2. In cases where surgery is indicated, the cardiologist should advise the patient as to who is the best surgeon for his condition. This second function is increasingly important because of the new surgical techniques which can now repair or alleviate many heart conditions.

As one cardiologist said: "The cardiologist who recommends you to a cardiac surgeon must know the answers to a number of specific questions about that surgeon. If he does not, then you may rightly ask him on what basis he is recommending the surgeon. If he does not answer you or brushes your question aside, persist with it. If he continues to ignore it, then you should see another cardiologist." (See heart surgery section for the most vital questions to ask regarding heart surgery.)

Besides ignoring your questions, are there any other signals from your cardiologist that might indicate that he or she is not of superior quality? A cardiologist answers: "Obviously if he hasn't passed his board certification for internal medicine and his cardiology sub-specialty boards this is a bad sign, but I think another bad sign is if he orders a battery of tests for you without first getting your full medical history. These tests may be very expensive and all of them may not be necessary. The cardiologist should be tailoring his tests to your specific problem."

The noninvasive tests that can now give accurate assessments of your heart's condition include the Holter ECG (this is a 24-hour electro-cardiographic monitoring of your heart); the stress ECG, which shows the heart's action when exercised; the echogram, which produces an ultrasound image of the heart; the thallium-201 radionuclide perfusion scan, which also images the heart. There is also heart catheter-ization, which is invasive. These tests should only be used when in-dicated and not just to collect a wide assortment of data.

The cardiologists listed here are outstanding consulting cardiol-ogists. They do not, as a rule, do primary care but rather act as consultants for the more difficult problems. Says one cardiologist: "If you have a relatively common problem, such as an uneventful recovery from a heart attack or uncomplicated angina, a general in-ternist with a subspecialty in cardiology may often be able to handle this. However, if there is a more serious situation, consulting with a cardiologist is recommended."

Almost all cardiologists practice general cardiology. However, in some instances those cardiologists known for special interests or spe-cial contributions in specific heart problems are so noted.

CARDIOLOGISTS

Dr. Robert J. Adolph
University of Cincinnati Medical School
Cincinnati, Ohio 45267

Professor of internal medicine.

Dr. Eugene Braunwald
Peter Bent Brigham Hospital
721 Huntington Avenue
Boston, Massachusetts 02115

Hersey professor of medicine, Harvard.

Dr. Lawrence S. Cohen
Yale–New Haven Hospital
333 Cedar Street
New Haven, Connecticut 06510

Professor of medicine.

Dr. Elliott Corday
University of California at Los Angeles Medical Center
Los Angeles, California 90024

Clinical professor of medicine.

Dr. Ernest Craige
338 Clinical Sciences Building
University of North Carolina Medical School
Chapel Hill, North Carolina 27514
Professor of medicine.

Dr. J. Michael Criley
University of California at Los Angeles–Harbor General Hospital
1000 West Carson Street
Torrance, California 90509

Dr. Roman DeSanctis
Massachusetts General Hospital
Boston, Massachusetts 02114
Professor of medicine, Harvard.

Dr. Joseph T. Doyle
Albany Medical College
Albany, New York 12208
Professor of medicine and head of cardiology.

Dr. Charles Fisch (rhythm abnormalities)
University of Indiana Medical Center
Indianapolis, Indiana 46202
Professor of medicine; director, division of cardiovascular medicine.

Dr. Allan Freidlich
Cardiac Unit
Massachusetts General Hospital
Boston, Massachusetts 02114
Associate clinical professor of medicine, Harvard.

Dr. Peter Gazes
Medical University of South Carolina
College of Medicine
Charleston, South Carolina 29403
Professor of medicine.

Dr. Michael S. Gordon
University of Miami Medical School
Biscayne Annex
Miami, Florida 33152
Associate professor of medicine, Miami.

Dr. Richard Gorlin
Mt. Sinai Hospital
100th Street and Fifth Avenue
New York, New York 10029
Professor and chairman, department of medicine.

Dr. David G. Greene
Buffalo General Hospital
100 High Street
Buffalo, New York 14203
Professor of medicine, State University of New York at Buffalo.

Dr. Rolf Gunnar
Loyola University Medical School
2160 South First Avenue
Maywood, Illinois 60153
Chairman, division of cardiology.

Dr. Robert Hall
Texas Heart Institute
6621 Fannin Street
Houston, Texas 77030
Clinical professor of medicine, Baylor; medical director of the Texas Heart Institute.

Dr. E. W. Hancock
Stanford University Hospital
Stanford, California 94305
Professor of medicine.

Dr. W. Proctor Harvey
Georgetown University Hospital
3800 Reservoir Road, NW
Washington, District of Columbia 20007
Professor of medicine.

Dr. J. O'Neal Humphries
Johns Hopkins Hospital
Baltimore, Maryland 21205

Professor of medicine.

Dr. J. Willis Hurst
Emory University Hospital
Atlanta, Georgia 30322

Professor and chairman, department of medicine.

Dr. Adolph Hutter, Jr.
Cardiac Unit
Massachusetts General Hospital
Boston, Massachusetts 02114

Associate professor of medicine, Harvard.

Dr. Albert A. Kattus, Jr.
Department of Medicine
University of California at Los Angeles Medical Center
Los Angeles, California 90024

Professor of medicine.

Dr. Thomas Killip
Henry Ford Hospital
Detroit, Michigan 48238

Chief of cardiology.

Dr. Charles E. Kossmann
University of Tennessee Medical School
951 Court
Memphis, Tennessee 38163

Professor of medicine.

Dr. William Likoff
Hahnemann Medical College
245 North 15th Street
Philadelphia, Pennsylvania 19102

Professor of medicine.

Dr. Bruce Logue
Emory University Clinic
1365 Clifton Road, NE
Atlanta, Georgia 30322

Professor of medicine.

Dr. Bernard Lown (rhythm abnormalities)
Peter Bent Brigham Hospital
Boston, Massachusetts 02115

Professor of medicine, Harvard.

Dr. Henry McIntosh
Watson Clinic
1600 Lakeland Hills Boulevard
Lakeland, Florida 33802

Dr. Frank I. Marcus
University of Arizona Health Science Center
Tucson, Arizona 85724

Professor of medicine and chief of cardiology.

Dr. Raymond D. Pruitt
Mayo Clinic
Rochester, Minnesota 55901

Dr. Charles E. Rackley
University of Alabama Medical Center
University Station
Birmingham, Alabama 35294

Professor of medicine.

Dr. Elliot Rapaport
University of California Medical Center
San Francisco, California 94143

Professor of medicine; director, cardiopulmonary unit, San Francisco General Hospital.

Dr. Richard O. Russell, Jr.
University of Alabama Medical
Center
Birmingham, Alabama 35233

Professor of medicine.

Dr. Robert Schlant
Emory University Hospital
Atlanta, Georgia 30322

Professor of medicine.

Dr. Arthur Selzer
Presbyterian Hospital Pacific
Medical Center
San Francisco, California 94120

*Clinical professor of medicine,
Stanford.*

Dr. W. Jape Taylor
University of Florida
J. H. Miller Health Center
Gainesville, Florida 32610

Professor of medicine.

Dr. Andrew G. Wallace
Duke University Medical Center
Durham, North Carolina 27710

*Professor of medicine;
chief of cardiology.*

Dr. James V. Warren
University Hospital
Columbus, Ohio 43210

*Professor and chairman,
department of medicine, Ohio State.*

Dr. Arnold M. Weissler
Wayne State University School of
Medicine
540 East Canfield Avenue
Detroit, Michigan 48201

*Professor and chairman, department
of internal medicine.*

Dr. A. Calhoun Witham
Medical College of Georgia
1120 15th Street
Augusta, Georgia 30901

Professor of medicine.

Dr. Paul N. Yu
University of Rochester
601 Elmwood Avenue
Rochester, New York 14642

*Sarah McCort Ward professor of
medicine.*

Dr. Peter Yurchak
Cardiac Unit
Massachusetts General Hospital
Boston, Massachusetts 02114

*Associate professor of medicine,
Harvard.*

Heart Surgeons

Although almost every major hospital in the country has a cardiac surgery team, there are few that are backed up by the excellent support teams required for this intricate and highly specialized kind of surgery.

Because most congenital heart defects are now treated by heart surgeons when the patients are very young, the heart surgery performed on adults is primarily for acquired heart problems. The major areas are valve repair and replacement surgery, cardiac aneurysm, constrictive pericarditis (when the sac around the heart interferes with the work of the heart), and the most controversial heart procedure, the coronary by-pass, which is performed on 100,000 Americans a year.

The coronary by-pass is a procedure in which veins (usually taken from the leg) are grafted onto the heart to by-pass the existing heart arteries which are failing because of blockages caused by arteriosclerosis. The arteriosclerosis in turn causes angina pectoris, a serious and painful heart condition. The by-pass operation remains controversial because there is no absolute proof that, once done, the operation guarantees the patient will live longer than he would have if he had not had the operation. However, interviews with a number of leading specialists, both cardiologists and cardiac surgeons, have revealed these generally accepted guidelines as to when coronary by-pass surgery may be indicated:

1. For patients with severe, limiting angina that alters their way of life and when the angina persists despite medication.

2. When there is a very high grade narrowing of the left main coronary artery. This can be detected by a thorough examination of the heart. It is believed that coronary by-pass in these cases may be helpful in prolonging the patient's life.

3. For persons with severe coronary disease, such as triple vessel disease.

4. For patients with unstable or rapidly progressive angina that requires hospitalization and causes changes on their electrocardiogram.

When may the by-pass *not* be advisable?

1. In people with mild, stable angina; i.e., infrequent pain that is controlled by medication.

2. In post–heart attack patients who are without symptoms after the heart attack.

It is well to keep these criteria in mind because of the overzealousness of some cardiac surgeons to operate when the indications are minimal. In part this is caused by federal policy. As part of a move to decrease medical costs, the federal government will no longer reimburse hospitals with cardiac units if they do less than 200 heart operations a year. (Massachusetts General, for example, does 1,100 heart operations a year.)

Although the idea behind this is to close down those centers which were not performing enough heart operations to justify their existence and cost, it has led to quite another problem. One cardiologist remarked: "What has happened is that many of the smaller cardiac surgery centers who really don't have enough patients in their local population for 200 heart operations a year are lowering the indications for the by-pass operation and giving it to people who really should not have it. I think eventually the trend will be towards the major centers doing these complicated procedures, but for now I think patients should be very careful about their advice for coronary surgery."

What steps can you take to insure you get the best advice about coronary by-pass? You should make certain that at least one of the cardiologists you consult is not associated with a heart surgeon and you should seek a second opinion, especially if you are at all uneasy about the diagnosis. If the heart surgery is advisable, you must ask hard questions of the surgeon and of the cardiologist. You should ask:

1. How many heart operations does the surgeon do each week? He should do several because repetition of the same procedure gives him and his team the knowledge and experience to better handle any complications.

2. What is the surgeon's patency rate? The patency rate is the rate at which the new by-passes he grafts to the heart remain open. The patency rate is determined by postoperative angiograms. If his patency rate is 85 to 90 percent, that is good. If the surgeon does not give you an answer, walk out. If the cardiologist who recommends him is not sure, ask why he is recommending the surgeon in the first place.

3. What are the surgeon's survival statistics? They should be better than 95 percent. The best centers have 98 to 99 percent in elective cases.

4. What is his peri-infarction rate (the rate of heart attacks during surgery)? Some patients have heart attacks (infarctions) on the operating table. They are usually not serious, and heart muscle damage is minor. However, a rate of 30 percent is very high. A rate of 10 percent is acceptable. Again, if the answers are vague or not forthcoming, see someone else.

5. What is the average number of grafts (by-passes) he places in the heart? If he replaces just one artery during the operation, that is

considered too low. A replacement of eight is considered too high. An average of three is considered good.

It cannot be too strongly stated: You must ask and demand answers. The patency rate is vital, of course. If the arteries shut down a few months after they've been grafted, then the operation has failed. As noted, in the best centers the patency rate is above 90 percent, but there are some with a rate as low as 69 percent. There are, however, many smaller cardiac centers in the country that have very acceptable heart surgery statistics. As one prominent cardiac surgeon noted: "It is very clear from all I have seen that you get very different results in heart surgery depending on where you go." The same is true of all surgery.

Below are listed some of the best cardiac surgeons in the country. They are known and selected for the very successes that were emphasized here, and for the added fact of their exceptional support teams and the wide experience they have in this field. All of the surgeons listed here have made their own unique contributions to heart surgery, and all still perform the full range of adult surgical procedures. One individual is singled out for his heart transplant work because he is getting the best results in the world. It should be noted, however, that heart transplantation is not perfected and remains a last measure when all other avenues have failed.

CARDIAC SURGEONS

Dr. W. Gerald Austen
Massachusetts General Hospital
Boston, Massachusetts 02114

Edward D. Churchill professor of surgery, Harvard.

Dr. Mortimer J. Buckley
Massachusetts General Hospital
Boston, Massachusetts 02114

Professor of surgery, Harvard.

Dr. John J. Collins, Jr.
Peter Bent Brigham Hospital
Boston, Massachusetts 02115

Professor of surgery, Harvard.

Dr. Denton Cooley
Texas Heart Institute
6621 Fannin Street
Houston, Texas 77030

He handles an enormous caseload, upward of twenty heart procedures a day.

Dr. Donald B. Effler
St. Joseph's Hospital
Syracuse, New York 13203

Formerly with the Cleveland Clinic; pioneered work in the coronary bypass.

Dr. Dudley Johnson
3112 West Highland Boulevard
Milwaukee, Wisconsin 53208

Another pioneer in coronary by-pass surgery; associate clinical professor of thoracic and cardiovascular surgery, Wisconsin Medical College.

Dr. John W. Kirklin
University of Alabama Medical Center
University Station
Birmingham, Alabama 35294

Chairman, department of surgery.

Dr. Nicholas Kouchoukos
University of Alabama Medical Center
University Station
Birmingham, Alabama 35294

Professor of surgery.

Dr. Floyd D. Loop
Cleveland Clinic
9500 Euclid Avenue
Cleveland, Ohio 44106

Chairman, department of cardio-thoracic surgery.

Dr. Richard Lower
Medical College of Virginia
Richmond, Virginia 23298

Professor and chairman, division of thoracic and cardiac surgery.

Dr. Dwight C. McGoon
Mayo Clinic
200 First Street, SW
Rochester, Minnesota 55901

Professor of surgery, Mayo Graduate School.

Dr. James R. Malm
161 Fort Washington Avenue
New York, New York 10032

Professor of clinical surgery, Columbia.

Dr. David C. Sabiston, Jr.
Duke Medical Center
Durham, North Carolina 27710

Professor and chairman, department of surgery.

Dr. Norman Shumway (transplant)
Stanford University Hospital
Stanford, California 94305

Chairman, department of cardiovascular surgery; has compiled the best results in heart transplant surgery.

Dr. Frank C. Spencer
New York University Medical Center
566 First Avenue
New York, New York 11016

Professor and chairman, department of surgery, New York University.

Dr. Albert Starr
University of Oregon Health Sciences Center
Portland, Oregon 97201

Professor of surgery; chief of cardiopulmonary surgery.

Hypertension Specialists

High blood pressure is perhaps the serious disorder easiest to diagnose and, in cases of only mildly elevated hypertension, one of the easiest to treat. Dietary salt restriction and weight loss sometimes reduce blood pressure levels to normal. However, in cases of serious or "malignant" hypertension the management of that disorder is difficult and sometimes exceedingly complex. It is also vital. In cases of malignant hypertension many people die within two years of kidney dysfunction, heart disease, or stroke.

What is hypertension? What defines it? There is no general agreement that a reading of 140 (systolic) over 90 (diastolic) means high blood pressure. This is considered borderline. However, readings of 160 (systolic) over 95 (diastolic) are generally regarded as evidence of hypertension that needs to be treated. This is also the standard accepted by the World Health Organization. These are the general categories of hypertension:

Diastolic Reading	*Type of Hypertension*
90–104	Mild (both non-drug and drug approaches as well as dietary changes are prescribed)
105–115	Moderate (dietary and drug approaches are usually used)
115 and above	Severe hypertension requiring immediate and expert medical attention.

What will a specialized hypertension clinic offer?

1. It will do a full diagnostic study including, when needed, kidney angiograms as well as many other tests. Also an expert who knows how to interpret the findings will be present.

2. Full patient education on all the aspects of your disorder will be made available. In hypertension, the patient's own care of himself is vital.

3. The best clinics call their clients to make certain they are taking care of themselves and remind them to come in for another visit. Because hypertension is often symptomless, many people tend to disregard their own self-treatment.

4. The best centers have at their disposal newer investigative drugs for those patients who do not respond to conventional therapies and

who are severely hypertensive. Virtually all cases of hypertension can be controlled if skillfully and expertly managed.

What are signs of inadequate hypertension management?

1. If your blood pressure is not brought under control, your kidney function may deteriorate and you may have other complications indicating that your management is not effective.

2. If major side effects of hypertensive drugs, such as muscle weakness, sexual dysfunction, drowsiness, and the like continue, you should consult a specialist.

3. Also, hypertensive women should be warned not to take the oral contraceptive pill, which can aggravate hypertension. Some doctors are not aware of this.

The following are some of the most outstanding hypertension specialists in the country. All of them are directly affiliated with a hypertension center at a hospital. This is important because full diagnostic workups for severely hypertensive patients are required and in many cases hospitalization is also required.

HYPERTENSION SPECIALISTS

Dr. John R. Caldwell
Henry Ford Hospital
Detroit, Michigan 48202

Associate professor of internal medicine, University of Michigan.

Dr. Aram V. Chobanian
Boston University Medical Center
80 East Concord Street
Boston, Massachusetts 02118

Professor of medicine, director of the Cardiovascular Institute at the Boston University Medical School.

Dr. Charles L. Curry
Howard University Hospital
Washington, District of Columbia 20060

Professor of medicine; director, division of cardiovascular diseases.

Dr. Harriet Dustan
University of Alabama Medical Center
Birmingham, Alabama 35233

Professor of medicine.

Dr. Karl Engleman
Hospital of the University of Pennsylvania
3400 Spruce Street
Philadelphia, Pennsylvania 19104

Associate professor of medicine and pharmacology; chief, hypertension section.

Dr. Edward D. Frohlich
Ochsner Clinic
New Orleans, Louisiana 70121

Director of the division of hypertensive diseases.

Dr. Ray W. Gifford, Jr.
Department of Hypertension and
Nephrology
Cleveland Clinic
Cleveland, Ohio 44106

Head of the department.

Dr. J. Caulie Gunnells, Jr.
Duke Medical Center
Durham, North Carolina 27710

Professor of medicine.

Dr. Roger Hickler
Worcester City Hospital
Worcester, Massachusetts 01610

Professor of medicine,
University of Massachusetts Medical
School.

Dr. John Hollifield
Hypertension Clinic
Vanderbilt Medical Center
Nashville, Tennessee 37232

Clinical director of the hypertension
clinic.

Dr. Harold Itskovitz
Milwaukee County General Hospital
Milwaukee, Wisconsin 53226

Professor of medicine, chief of
hypertension service, Medical
College of Wisconsin.

Dr. Stevo Julius
University of Michigan Medical
Center
Ann Arbor, Michigan 48104

Professor of medicine.

Dr. Norman M. Kaplan
Southwestern Medical School
5323 Harry Hines Boulevard
Dallas, Texas 75235

Professor of internal medicine.

Dr. Walter Kirkendall
Department of Medicine
University of Texas Medical School
Houston, Texas 77030

Professor of medicine.

Dr. Herbert Langford
University of Mississippi
2500 North State Street
Jackson, Mississippi 39216

Director of the hypertension unit.

Dr. John H. Laragh
New York Hospital–Cornell
Medical Center
525 East 68th Street
New York, New York 10021

Master professor of medicine;
director of the hypertension and
cardiovascular center, Cornell
Medical School.

Dr. F. Gilbert McMahon
1430 Tulane Avenue
New Orleans, Louisiana 70112

Professor of medicine, Tulane.

Dr. Morton H. Maxwell
Cedars-Sinai Medical Center
8700 Beverly Boulevard
Los Angeles, California 90048

Director, hypertension service;
clinical professor of medicine,
University of California at Los
Angeles.

Dr. James C. Melby
750 Harrison Avenue
Boston, Massachusetts 02118

Professor of medicine, Boston
University.

Dr. John A. Oates
Vanderbilt Medical Center
Nashville, Tennessee 37232

Professor of internal medicine and pharmacology.

Dr. Gaddo Onesti
Hahnemann Medical College and Hospital
230 North Broad Street
Philadelphia, Pennsylvania 19102

Professor of medicine.

Dr. Lot B. Page
2000 Washington Street
Newton Lower Falls, Massachusetts 02162

Chief of medicine, Newton-Wellesley Hospital.

Dr. Sheldon G. Sheps
Mayo Clinic
Rochester, Minnesota 55901

Associate professor of medicine, Mayo.

Dr. Cameron G. Strong
Mayo Clinic
Rochester, Minnesota 55901

Professor of medicine, Mayo.

Dr. Louis Tobian
Hypertension Clinic
University of Minnesota Hospitals
Minneapolis, Minnesota 55455

Director of hypertension clinic.

Dr. Donald Vidt
Cleveland Clinic
Cleveland, Ohio 44106

Head of the clinical section on hypertension and nephrology.

Dr. James W. Woods, Jr.
University of North Carolina
Medical School
Chapel Hill, North Carolina 27514

Professor of medicine.

Dr. Andrew Zweifler
University of Michigan Medical Center
Ann Arbor, Michigan 48104

Professor of internal medicine.

Lipid Disorder Specialists

Two lipids found in the bloodstream—cholesterol and triglycerides—are considered important risk factors in heart and cerebrovascular disease, although elevated cholesterol is regarded as the more significant problem.

Because of their suspected role in these diseases, blood lipids are coming under increasing study. General internists and endocrinologists look into the causes and possible cures for a high level of lipids in the bloodstream, although the field is closely allied with cardiology and neurology.

In some instances, high levels of cholesterol and triglycerides can be reduced by dietary changes. However, in some individuals there is a genetic tendency to have excessively high levels of cholesterol and dietary changes have little effect. High triglyceride levels and high blood sugar levels—a form of adult onset diabetes—often coexist. "In many of these cases the management is extremely complex," one lipid specialist remarked, "because by treating the hyperlipemia incorrectly, you can actually make the patient's overall condition worse, not better. You treat different types of the disorder very differently."

Physicians disagree over what constitutes high cholesterol levels. Some regard any reading above 220 mg. as excessive, others regard anything above 190 mg. as excessive. However, they generally all agree that cholesterol above 250 mg. (it can be found through a simple blood test) is excessively high and should be treated in some way. Treatment of hyperlipemia often includes drugs as well as dietary changes.

Listed are a number of individuals noted for their interest in lipid disorders as they affect children and adults. Some are endocrinologists, others are cardiologists. Many are primarily researchers but have a clinical interest in some patients or can serve as a referral base for people. Also included are several lipid research centers funded by the National Institutes of Health. Although private patient access to the National Institutes of Health research centers is very unlikely, several of the physicians listed under these centers do see private patients and can also serve as a referral base. Those individuals who are primarily researchers are so noted, as are those who do more patient care.

LIPID DISORDER SPECIALISTS

Dr. Francois Abboud, director
Dr. Mark Armstrong
Dr. Helmut Schrott
Dr. Arthur Spector
Lipid Research Clinic
University of Iowa Hospitals
Iowa City, Iowa 52240

This is a National Institutes of Health lipid research center. Dr. Schrott does patient care.

Dr. Edwin Bierman
University of Washington Medical School
Seattle, Washington 98195

Professor of medicine. Patients and referrals.

Dr. Reagan H. Bradford, director
Lipid Research Center
Oklahoma Medical Research Foundation
Oklahoma City, Oklahoma 73104

Part of the National Institutes of Health lipid research study. Referral and clinical care.

Dr. Michael Brown
Dr. Joseph Goldstein
Dr. David Bilheimer
Southwestern Medical School
Dallas, Texas 75235

Doctors Brown and Goldstein do lipid research. Dr. Bilheimer does clinical care.

Dr. Brian Brewer
Dr. Thomas Bersot
Metabolic Disease Branch
National Institutes of Health
Building 10
Bethesda, Maryland 20014

Like all National Institutes of Health care, it is free. However, patients require referrals from their physicians and they must meet the National Institutes of Health research protocols.

Dr. William E. Connor
Department of Internal Medicine
University of Oregon School for
Health Sciences
Portland, Oregon 97201

Professor of internal medicine.

Dr. Oscar B. Crofford
Vanderbilt Medical Center
Nashville, Tennessee 37232

Special emphasis on patients having both diabetes and lipid disorders.

Dr. Howard Eder
Albert Einstein Medical School
Bronx, New York 10461

Dr. Eder has an active clinical practice.

Dr. John Farquhar, director
Heart Disease Prevention Center
Stanford Medical Center
Stanford, California 94305

A strong emphasis on behavior changes to prevent heart disease.

Dr. Ivan Frantz, director
Dr. Donald Hunninghake,
co-director
University of Minnesota Medical
School
Minneapolis, Minnesota 55455

Part of the National Institutes of Health lipid research study. Referral and clinical work.

Dr. Charles J. Glueck
Lipid Research Center
University of Cincinnati Medical
School
Cincinnati, Ohio 45267

Part of the National Institutes of Health study. Referral and private patients.

Dr. DeWitt Goodman
Dr. Robert Glickman
Hyperlipemia Clinic
Columbia-Presbyterian Medical
Center
New York, New York 10032

Private patients.

Dr. William Insull, director
Dr. Antonio M. Gotto, co-director
Lipid Research Center
Baylor College of Medicine
Houston, Texas 77030

Part of the National Institutes of Health study. Referral and some private patients.

Dr. Robert H. Knopp
Lipid Research Center
University of Washington Medical
School
Seattle, Washington 98195

Part of the National Institutes of Health study. Patients and referral.

Dr. Peter O. Kwiterovich
Lipid Research Center
Johns Hopkins Medical School
Baltimore, Maryland 21205

Part of the National Institutes of Health study. Patients and referrals.

Dr. John LaRosa
Lipid Research Center
George Washington University Hospital
Washington, District of Columbia 20037

Part of the National Institutes of Health study. Patients and referrals.

Dr. J. Alick Little
Lipid Research Center
Toronto General Hospital
Toronto, Ontario
Canada M5G 1L7

Part of the National Institutes of Health study. Patients and referral.

Dr. Simeon Margolis
The Johns Hopkins Hospital
Baltimore, Maryland 21205

Professor of medicine. Patients and referrals.

Dr. Gustav Schonfeld
Washington University Medical School
St. Louis, Missouri 63110

Part of the National Institutes of Health study. Patients and referrals.

Dr. John Turner, director
Dr. Daniel Steinberg, co-director
University of California Medical School
La Jolla, California 92037

Part of the National Institutes of Health study. Patients and referrals.

Peripheral Vascular Disease Specialists

Peripheral vascular disease specialists treat vascular problems that occur outside of the heart and the brain. Although many people suffer some form of peripheral vascular disease, there are only two major medical clinics in the country that deal with the medical aspects of this disorder—the *Mayo Clinic* and the *Cleveland Clinic*. Furthermore, there are very few internists in the U.S. who devote their entire practice to peripheral vascular disease. As one peripheral vascular disease specialist remarked: "It is a scandal in one sense because many people are in need of treatment for vascular disease and there are so few specialists other than surgeons to treat them. At our clinic we are treating an enormous number of patients simply because there are so few places to go." Another vascular medical specialist noted: "The art of managing peripheral vascular disease is much neglected."

There are a number of vascular diseases, but by far the most common is arteriosclerosis, which can cause claudication or pain in leg arteries during exercise. Other vascular diseases include varicose veins, inflammatory diseases of the vascular system, aneurysms, venous thrombophlebitis (commonly known as phlebitis), and other clotting problems, as well as a number of rarer vascular diseases.

There are a number of treatments available for vascular disease, including drug treatment and surgery. In fact, because of the absence of a large number of vascular disease specialists, many vascular surgeons have assumed nonsurgical treatment of some patients. Some vascular surgeons, in fact, have devised methods of diagnosis that greatly improved previous methods. Please consult the vascular surgery list also.

Another major cause of vascular disease is diabetes. The damage to the lower extremities, particularly the feet, from diabetes' effect on the vascular system can be extremely serious. New surgical techniques have been devised in recent years to revascularize these areas when diabetes has damaged or destroyed them, but there are also some nonsurgical approaches to diabetic vascular problems.

Below are listed outstanding vascular disease specialists at both the Mayo Clinic and the Cleveland Clinic. There are also several other individual doctors noted for their expertise in this specialty.

PERIPHERAL VASCULAR DISEASE SPECIALISTS

Dr. John Fairbairn
Dr. John Joyce
Dr. John L. Juergens
Dr. John A. Spittell
Mayo Clinic
Rochester, Minnesota 55901

All are considered excellent vascular disease specialists.

Dr. Jesse R. Young
Dr. Victor G. deWolfe
Dr. William Raschhaupt
Cleveland Clinic
Cleveland, Ohio 44106

Dr. Young is the chairman of the peripheral vascular unit.

Dr. Donald J. Breslin
Lahey Clinic
605 Commonwealth Avenue
Boston, Massachusetts 02215

Dr. Jay D. Coffman
University Hospital
Boston, Massachusetts 02118

Professor of medicine, Boston University; head of the peripheral vascular unit.

Dr. William Foley
441 East 68th Street
New York, New York 10021

Associate professor of medicine, Cornell.

Dr. Victor Gurewich
300 Mt. Auburn Street
Cambridge, Massachusetts 02138

Assistant clinical professor of medicine, Harvard; director of the vascular lab, St. Elizabeth's Hospital, Brighton.

Dr. Orville Horwitz
Franklin Medical Building
829 Spruce Street
Philadelphia, Pennsylvania 19107

Professor of medicine and pharmacology, University of Pennsylvania.

Dr. Irwin J. Schatz
University of Hawaii Medical School
Honolulu, Hawaii 96813

Professor and chairman, department of medicine.

Dr. Travis Winsor
Memorial Heart Research Foundation
4041 Wilshire Boulevard
Los Angeles, California 90010

Clinical professor of medicine, Southern California Medical School.

Dr. Kenneth Woolling
1815 North Capitol Avenue
Suite 306
Indianapolis, Indiana 46202

Director, coronary care unit and cardiovascular laboratory, Methodist Hospital.

Dr. Irving S. Wright
450 East 69th Street
New York, New York 10021

Emeritus professor of clinical medicine, Cornell.

Peripheral Vascular Surgeons

Peripheral vascular surgeons operate on the vascular system other than the heart and the brain. As a general rule, when vascular problems are mild they are treated medically, but in the intermediate stages of the disease, vascular surgery can repair and restructure significant parts of the vascular system. Although peripheral vascular surgeons perform the full range of vascular surgery, many have special interests in different vascular problems. Furthermore, because there are so few internal medicine specialists who specialize in vascular disease, many vascular surgeons are also noted for their diagnostic techniques and for their medical treatment of vascular disease. The following are the major special interests of vascular surgeons:

Carotid artery surgery. The two carotid arteries which carry blood to the head through the neck become narrowed in many people because of arteriosclerosis. Some vascular surgeons have a special interest in carotid artery surgery, which can fully or nearly fully reopen the carotid arteries and allow the blood flow to the brain, face, and head to resume.

Revascularization. Because of the damage diabetes inflicts on the vascular system, some diabetics lose blood flow to their lower legs and feet. Although all vascular surgeons do considerable revascularization surgery, some have a special interest in this area because of the large number of diabetics in the country.

Aneurysms. An aneurysm is a ballooning of an artery often caused by a congenital weakness. Aortic aneurysms are probably the most serious aneurysms outside of the brain because of the enormous blood flow through the aorta. Some vascular surgeons have a special interest in aneurysm and aortic aneurysm surgery.

Vein grafts. Vein problems, including varicose veins and phlebitis, may require vein graft surgery in which part of the venous system is restructured to permit more normal blood flow.

Iliac surgery. The iliac arteries are the main branch arteries leading from the aorta to the legs. Many conditions can require surgery, such as aneurysms, or arteriosclerosis, which can also cause claudication.

Claudication. This is a condition in which arteries are blocked or narrowed, causing severe and often debilitating pain, particularly in the legs.

Renal hypertension. The narrowing of the major artery leading from the kidney can cause high blood pressure and can require surgery to restore normal blood flow and normal blood pressure. Some urologists also have a special interest in this area.

Diagnosis. Some vascular surgeons are noted for their diagnostic work in vascular disease. They are so identified.

Some of the vascular surgeons listed do not have special interests or special areas of concentration. Some of the vascular surgeons are general surgeons who have specialized in vascular work, or are thoracic surgeons who specialize in vascular surgery and, in some cases, cardiovascular surgery.

PERIPHERAL VASCULAR SURGEONS

Dr. Wiley F. Barker (aortic and iliac)
University of California at Los Angeles Medical Center
Los Angeles, California 90024

Professor of surgery.

Dr. Robert W. Barnes
Medical College of Virginia
Richmond, Virginia 23298

Professor of surgery.

Dr. John J. Bergan
251 East Chicago Avenue
Chicago, Illinois 60611

*Professor of surgery at
Northwestern University Medical
School. Known for his diagnostic
techniques.*

Dr. Philip Bernatz (aortic and iliac)
Mayo Clinic
Rochester, Minnesota 55901

Professor of surgery at Mayo.

Dr. John J. Cranley
Good Samaritan Hospital
Cincinnati, Ohio 45220

*Associate clinical professor of
surgery, University of Cincinnati.
Known for his diagnostic techniques.*

Dr. E. Stanley Crawford (chest and
abdominal aneurysms)
Baylor College of Medicine
Houston, Texas 77025

Professor of surgery.

Dr. W. Andrew Dale (vein grafts)
Vanderbilt Medical Center
Nashville, Tennessee 37232

Professor of surgery.

Dr. Clement R. Darling
(abdominal aortic aneurysms)
Massachusetts General Hospital
Boston, Massachusetts 02114

Professor of surgery, Harvard.

Dr. James A. DeWesse
(vein grafts)
Strong Memorial Hospital of the
University of Rochester
601 Elmwood Avenue
Rochester, New York 14642

Professor of cardio-thoracic surgery.

Dr. Sterling Edwards
(aortic surgery)
University of New Mexico
Medical School
Albuquerque, New Mexico 87106

*Professor and chairman,
department of surgery.*

Dr. Thomas J. Fogarty
(aortic surgery)
770 Welch Road
Suite 201
Palo Alto, California 94304

*Associate professor of surgery,
Stanford.*

Dr. William Fry (renal
hypertension)
Southwestern Medical School
Dallas, Texas 75235

*Professor and chairman, department
of surgery.*

Dr. Charles Hufnagel (aortic
aneurysms)
Georgetown University Hospital
3800 Reservoir Road, NW
Washington, District of Columbia
20007

*Professor and chairman, department
of surgery.*

Dr. Anthony M. Imparato
(carotid artery)
New York University Medical
Center
566 First Avenue
New York, New York 10016

Professor of surgery.

Dr. Richard O. Kraft
St. Joseph's Mercy Hospital
Ann Arbor, Michigan 48104

*Clinical professor of surgery,
University of Michigan Medical
School.*

Dr. John Mannick
(revascularization of legs)
Peter Bent Brigham Hospital
Boston, Massachusetts 02115

Professor of surgery, Harvard.

Dr. Wesley Moore (carotid artery)
University of Arizona Health
Sciences Center
Tucson, Arizona 85724

Professor of surgery.

Dr. George C. Morris, Jr.
Baylor College of Medicine
Houston, Texas 77025

Professor of surgery.

Dr. Roger F. Smith
Henry Ford Hospital
Detroit, Michigan 48202

*Clinical professor of surgery,
University of Michigan Medical
School.*

Dr. Ronald J. Stoney
University of California Medical
Center
San Francisco, California 94143

Professor of medicine.

Dr. Eugene Strandness, Jr.
1959 NE Pacific Avenue
Seattle, Washington 98105

*Professor of surgery, University
of Washington Medical School.
Noted for his noninvasive diagnostic
techniques.*

Dr. Jesse E. Thompson (carotid
artery)
3600 Gaston Avenue
Suite 505
Dallas, Texas 75246

*Professor of surgery, Southwestern
Medical School.*

Dr. Edwin J. Wylie (carotid artery;
claudication; aneurysms)
University of California Medical
Center
350 Parnassus
San Francisco, California 94117

*Professor of surgery. Considered a
major figure in the advancement of
vascular surgery.*

Diseases of the Chest

Diseases of the Lung

Lung disease is epidemic and the major cause is cigarette smoking. Emphysema, chronic bronchitis, and lung cancer are the three major lung diseases caused by smoking and, as one pulmonary specialist said: "My only advice as to how to improve our statistics regarding lung diseases is to stop smoking. We simply can't do enough in many cases to ameliorate the symptoms once the disease has progressed."

Pulmonary specialists in many cases cannot reverse the trend of these lung diseases. Rather, they have an assortment of devices and treatment techniques to lessen symptoms and allow the patient to lead a more normal life. "We see many patients after their family doctors have given up on them," said the pulmonary specialist. "The doctors seemed relieved that we are treating the patient because these obstructive lung diseases are so difficult to handle. Also, we see patient after patient in which the standard procedures are not being used to alleviate symptoms."

What are some of the standard procedures used by lung specialists that are sometimes overlooked by nonspecialists?

1. In many cases infections are not treated or are not treated correctly.

2. Bronchodilators, which open air passageways to the lungs, are

often not used in treatment, thereby creating additional problems for the patient.

3. Respirators to aid breathing are often not used.

"What we do see, however," this same lung specialist remarked, "is the too frequent use of steroids (such as cortisone) in the treatment of emphysema and chronic bronchitis. These drugs are largely useless; they have only a very limited use in treatment because they do little good for the patient and because they have such serious side effects."

Lung specialists, unlike many other specialists, do not generally subspecialize. All lung specialists do respiration therapy, treat and manage chronic bronchitis, tuberculosis, emphysema, nonoperable lung cancer, sarcoidosis, and other pulmonary diseases, as well as treat patients who have had surgery for lung cancer.

However, some pulmonary specialists have a special interest or special expertise in certain disorders. Largely because of geography, some lung specialists have developed special expertise in *occupational lung diseases* such as black lung, brown lung, asbestosis, and other work-related lung disorders. In addition, some have special expertise in *thromboembolic diseases*—disorders that cause blood clots in the lung.

LUNG SPECIALISTS

Dr. Whitney W. Addington
Cook County Hospital
1825 West Harrison Street
Chicago, Illinois 60612

Head of pulmonary medicine, Cook County Hospital; assistant professor of medicine, Northwestern.

Dr. William H. Anderson
University of Louisville School of Medicine
Louisville, Kentucky 40232

Professor of medicine; director of cardiopulmonary laboratory, Harlan Memorial Hospital.

Dr. Wilmot C. Ball, Jr.
Johns Hopkins Hospital
Baltimore, Maryland 21205

Associate professor of medicine.

Dr. Joseph Bates
University of Arkansas Medical Center
Little Rock, Arkansas 72201

Professor of internal medicine and microbiology.

Dr. Leo Black
Mayo Clinic
Rochester, Minnesota 55901

Associate professor of medicine, Mayo.

Dr. Richard E. Brashear
University of Indiana Medical
Center
Indianapolis, Indiana 46202

*Director, division of pulmonary
medicine; professor of medicine.*

Dr. Dick D. Briggs, Jr.
University of Alabama Medical
Center
Birmingham, Alabama 35294

*Professor of medicine and director
of pulmonary medicine.*

Dr. Helen A. Dickie
University Hospital
Madison, Wisconsin 53706

*Professor of medicine; head,
pulmonary section, University of
Wisconsin Medical School.*

Dr. Matthew Divertie
Mayo Clinic
Rochester, Minnesota 55901

Professor of medicine, Mayo.

Dr. Ronald George
Louisiana State University Medical
School
510 East Stover Avenue
Shreveport, Louisiana 71130

*Head, pulmonary disease section;
professor of internal medicine.*

Dr. Leonard D. Hudson
Harborview Medical Center
Seattle, Washington 98101

*Professor of medicine, University of
Washington; chief of respiratory
disease division at Harborview.*

Dr. Roland Ingram
Peter Bent Brigham Hospital
Boston, Massachusetts 02115

*Chief of pulmonary medicine;
associate professor of medicine,
Harvard.*

Dr. Daniel E. Jenkins
Baylor College of Medicine
Houston, Texas 77025

Professor of medicine.

Dr. Sol Katz
Georgetown University Hospital
Washington, District of Columbia
20007

*Professor of medicine; director,
pulmonary disease section.*

Dr. Gerald Kerby
Kansas Medical Center
Kansas City, Kansas 66103

Associate professor of medicine.

Dr. Glen Lillington
University of California at Davis
Davis, California 95616

*Professor of medicine; head of
pulmonary medicine.*

Dr. John H. McClement
New York University Medical
School
550 First Avenue
New York, New York 10016

Professor of medicine.

Dr. Richard A. Matthay
Yale University Medical School
New Haven, Connecticut 06511

*Associate director, pulmonary
disease section.*

Dr. Robert L. Mayock
Hospital of the University of
Pennsylvania
3400 Spruce Street
Philadelphia, Pennsylvania 19104

Professor of medicine.

Dr. R. Drew Miller
Mayo Clinic
Rochester, Minnesota 55901

Professor of medicine at Mayo.

Dr. Kenneth M. Moser
(thromboembolic disorders)
University Hospital
225 West Dickinson
San Diego, California 92103

*Professor of medicine and director
of pulmonary division.*

Dr. John F. Murray
University of California Medical
Center
San Francisco, California 94143

Professor of medicine.

Dr. Thomas A. Neff
University of Colorado Medical
Center
Denver, Colorado 80220

*Chief, pulmonary disease section,
Denver General Hospital.*

Dr. Donald Olson
Portland Clinic
800 SW 13th
Portland, Oregon 97205

Dr. Thomas L. Petty
University of Colorado Medical
Center
Denver, Colorado 80220

Professor of medicine at Colorado.

Dr. Alan K. Pierce
Southwestern Medical School
5323 Harry Hines Boulevard
Dallas, Texas 75235

Professor of medicine.

Dr. Attilio D. Renzetti, Jr.
University of Utah Medical Center
50 North Medical Center Drive
Salt Lake City, Utah 84132

Professor of medicine.

Dr. Robert M. Rogers
University of Oklahoma Health
Sciences Center
Oklahoma City, Oklahoma 73109

*Professor of medicine and chief of
pulmonary disease section.*

Dr. Joseph C. Ross
Medical University of South
Carolina
171 Ashley Avenue
Charleston, South Carolina 29401

*Professor and chairman, department
of medicine.*

Dr. William E. Ruth
Kansas Medical Center
Kansas City, Kansas 61103

*Professor of medicine and chief of
pulmonary disease section.*

Dr. Marvin A. Sackner
4300 Alton Road
Miami Beach, Florida 33140

Professor of medicine at Miami.

Dr. Jules R. Schwaber
Lahey Clinic
605 Commonwealth Avenue
Boston, Massachusetts 02215

*Clinical instructor in medicine at
Harvard.*

Dr. Robert M. Senior
Jewish Hospital
216 South Kingshighway
St. Louis, Missouri 63110

Director, division of pulmonary diseases, Jewish Hospital, and associate professor of medicine at Washington University School of Medicine.

Dr. Herbert O. Sieker
Duke Medical Center
Durham, North Carolina 27710

Professor of internal medicine.

Dr. James P. Smith
170 East 77th Street
New York, New York 10021

Associate clinical professor of medicine, Columbia.

Dr. Gordon L. Snider
University Hospital
75 East Newton Street
Boston, Massachusetts 02118

Professor of medicine at Boston University Medical School.

Dr. Myron Stein
Mt. Sinai General Hospital
8720 Beverly Boulevard
Los Angeles, California 90048

Dr. Paul Stevens
Baylor College of Medicine
Houston, Texas 77025

Chief of the pulmonary section, Baylor.

Dr. Alvin S. Teirstein
70 East 90th Street
New York, New York 10028

Clinical professor of medicine, Mt. Sinai Medical School.

Dr. John G. Weg
University of Michigan Medical Center
Ann Arbor, Michigan 48104

Professor of medicine; physician in charge of pulmonary division.

Dr. Hans Weill (occupational pulmonary disease)
1700 Perdido Street
New Orleans, Louisiana 70012

Professor of medicine, Tulane University.

Dr. Morton M. Ziskind
(occupational pulmonary disease)
1700 Perdido Street
New Orleans, Louisiana 70012

Professor of medicine, Tulane University.

Thoracic Surgeons

Because of the epidemic of lung cancer (it is the most common kind of terminal cancer in the U.S.), thoracic surgeons are performing more and more lung cancer surgery. Although the cure rate for lung cancer after surgery is improving, that statistic is misleading. The major reason why lung cancer patients are doing better statistically after surgery is because those who have a very poor prognosis are not operated on in the first place. "Many lung cancers are inoperable," one prominent thoracic surgeon remarked, "so at the very beginning we rule out a lot of people for surgery simply because we realize that they won't be helped by surgery. Perhaps a half of those patients diagnosed with lung cancer are actually operated on and the remainder are treated medically."

Thoracic surgeons perform other chest surgery besides lung cancer. Sometimes emphysema causes blisters on the lung which have to be removed surgically. Also, the esophagus is operated on by thoracic surgeons as well as general surgeons. It is an area of overlap in which different specialties do the same thing. The trachea is also surgically treated by thoracic surgeons.

Thoracic surgeons do subspecialize into two other areas, cardiac surgery and peripheral vascular surgery. Thoracic specialists who have subspecialized in these areas appear under those listings. The thoracic surgeons who appear in this list perform the full range of general thoracic surgery, including lung cancer, some surgery for infectious problems as well as esophageal and tracheal surgery. Largely because of the volume of lung cancer surgery, all of the surgeons who appear on this list have wide experience in lung cancer surgery.

Other special interests of thoracic surgeons include:

Tracheal reconstruction. Repair and reconstruction of the trachea (the windpipe) after injury or disease, such as tumors.

Esophagus. This can include cancer or hiatal hernia repair or other surgery on the esophagus, including cancer. The esophagus is the tube that carries food from the mouth to the stomach.

As noted, and it should be emphasized, *all* of the thoracic surgeons listed here perform the full range of general thoracic surgical procedures, but those with special interests in certain types of surgery are so noted.

THORACIC SURGEONS

Dr. Edward J. Beattie (lung cancer)
Memorial Hospital for Cancer and
Allied Diseases
1275 York Avenue
New York, New York 10021

*Chairman, department of surgery;
professor of surgery, Cornell
Medical School. A recognized lung
cancer authority.*

Dr. Philip E. Bernatz
Mayo Clinic
200 First Street, SW
Rochester, Minnesota 55901

Professor of surgery.

Dr. F. Henry Ellis, Jr. (esophagus)
Lahey Clinic
605 Commonwealth Avenue
Boston, Massachusetts 02215

Dr. Robert G. Ellison
Medical College of Georgia
Augusta, Georgia 30901

Professor of surgery and chief of the thoracic and cardiac surgery division.

Dr. Thomas B. Ferguson
4989 Barnes Hospital Plaza
St. Louis, Missouri 63110

Professor of clinical, thoracic, and cardiovascular surgery, Washington University Medical School.

Dr. Hermes Grillo
(tracheal reconstruction)
Massachusetts General Hospital
Boston, Massachusetts 02114

Professor of surgery, Harvard.

Dr. Clement A. Hiebert
321 Brackett Street
Portland, Maine 04102

Dr. Robert J. Jensik (lung cancer)
1725 West Harrison Street
Chicago, Illinois 60612

Clinical professor of surgery, Rush Medical College and University of Illinois Medical School. Special interest in lung cancer.

Dr. James Mark
Stanford Medical Center
Stanford, California 94305

Professor of surgery, head of thoracic surgery.

Dr. Martin F. McKneally (lung cancer)
Albany Medical College
Albany, New York 12208

Associate professor of surgery. Noted for his work in the immunologic response to lung cancer.

Dr. Nael Martini (lung cancer)
Memorial Hospital for Cancer and Allied Diseases
1275 York Avenue
New York, New York 10021

Chief of thoracic surgery.

Dr. Donald Mulder
University of California at Los Angeles Medical Center
Los Angeles, California 90024

Professor of surgery.

Dr. Donald L. Paulson (lung cancer)
653 Wadley Tower
Baylor Medical Plaza
3600 Gaston Avenue
Dallas, Texas 75246

Clinical professor of thoracic surgery, Southwestern Medical School.

Dr. W. Spencer Payne
Mayo Clinic
200 First Street, SW
Rochester, Minnesota 55901

Professor of surgery.

Dr. Joseph W. Peabody, Jr.
1234 19th Street, NW
Washington, District of Columbia 20036

Clinical assistant professor of surgery, Georgetown University Medical School.

Dr. F. Griffith Pearson
(tracheal reconstruction)
Toronto General Hospital
Toronto, Ontario
Canada M5G 1L7

Dr. Richard M. Peters
University of California Hospital
San Diego, California 92103

*Professor of surgery; chief of
thoracic surgery.*

Dr. J. Gordon Scannel
Massachusetts General Hospital
Boston, Massachusetts 02114

Professor of surgery, Harvard.

Dr. Will Camp Sealey
Duke Medical Center
Durham, North Carolina 27110

*Professor and chief of thoracic
surgery.*

Dr. E. Wayne Wilkins (esophagus
and lung)
Massachusetts General Hospital
Boston, Massachusetts 02114

*Associate professor of surgery,
Harvard.*

Dr. W. Glenn Young, Jr.
Duke Medical Center
Durham, North Carolina 27710

Professor of surgery.

Diseases of the Nervous System

Neurologists

A grim joke has for years made the rounds in medical circles that neurologists served two functions: First they diagnosed untreatable neurologic illnesses and then told the patient how long he or she had to live.

In some neurological illnesses this still holds true. However, in a number of other previously untreatable illnesses, including multiple sclerosis, myasthenia gravis, Parkinson's disease, and dementia, there are now treatments which can often ameliorate the patient's symptoms and in some cases cause a reversal of the disease. "There are good ways to manage patients even with incurable neurological disorders," one prominent neurologist remarked, "and by taking care of symptoms you can greatly improve the patient's life."

Some formerly incapacitating and fatal neurological illnesses are now responding very well to different treatments. Myasthenia gravis, for example (a neuromuscular disease which causes gradual weakening of the muscles), is responding well to both drug therapy and a surgical procedure called a thymectomy (removal of the thymus gland from the chest). In acute cases of this disease, a treatment called plasmapheresis is sometimes used and has reportedly lessened if not eliminated the symptoms of many patients. However, this treatment, which is used routinely in many blood disorders, remains a controversial treatment for myasthenia gravis. In multiple sclerosis, a disease which strikes young and middle-aged adults, there are treatments that can cause some of the symptoms to subside.

Dementia, or senile dementia, popularly believed to be caused by "hardening of the arteries," is in fact caused by a number of different conditions, many of which are treatable. Only one of the causes, and a rare one at that, is from cerebrovascular disease. Nutrition problems, vitamin B-12 deficiency, and tumors are but a few of the possible causes of this disorder.

Given the fact that many neurological disorders are complex and often baffling to non-neurologists, the question is when should consultation with specialists be sought? One neurologist says: "This can be readily divided into whether it is a problem where the diagnosis is known but the management is difficult, or whether it is for the diagnosis of an enigmatic disease. If the problem is an uncomplicated one, then numerous consultations are not needed and will probably confuse the patient more than help. But if it is complicated, then consultations may be important to accurately diagnose the illness because if it can be precisely diagnosed, there may be something we can do about it."

Like other specialists, neurologists tend to have special interests in various neurological disorders. Here are the general categories of neurologic special interests.

Cerebrovascular disease. This is the most common neurologic disorder and one of the most life-threatening. After heart disease and cancer, strokes are the nation's biggest killer. However, early detection and treatment of vascular disease can be of great benefit to patients. Another serious vascular disorder is cerebral aneurysm. Most are treated surgically by neurosurgeons, and others are treated medically.

Neuromuscular diseases. The muscle is the largest organ of the body yet there is no specialty which deals with it exclusively. The most common neuromuscular problem is inflammation, which causes a person's muscles to feel stiff and aching, as if he or she had done too much exercise the day before. It is like arthritis of the muscles. More serious and complex forms of neuromuscular disease include amyotrophic lateral sclerosis (Lou Gehrig's disease), the different types of muscular dystrophy, and myasthenia gravis. Some muscle disorders caused by toxins, such as arsenic and lead, are also classified as neuromuscular. Some of these neuromuscular diseases can be reversed, some can only have their symptoms ameliorated.

Viral diseases. Measles and polio are the most widely known neurological viral diseases. However, since the advent of measles vaccine, measles is usually benign except in rare cases, and polio is extremely rare today because of the Salk and Sabin vaccines. Encephalitis and a disease known as herpes zoster, which causes a skin disease known as shingles, are both among the more common neurological viral diseases.

Bacterial infections. The most common bacterial infections are the different types of meningitis.

Epilepsy. This seizure disorder, which can be caused by genetics or biochemistry, and in some cases by a head injury, can be controlled by drugs, but in some cases the management is complex. Also, there are surgical procedures that can control intractable epileptic seizures. Specialists in these neurosurgical techniques appear under neurosurgery.

Involuntary movement disorders. These include Parkinson's disease, tics, tremors, inherited ataxias, and dystonia.

Multiple sclerosis. The cause of this disease is unknown, but because it strikes a large number of people (sixty out of every 100,000) some neurologists have made the disease their subspecialty. In some cases, it is a very difficult disease to diagnose with absolute certainty.

Dementia. As noted, there are several different causes of this disorder, and if a correct diagnosis of the cause can be made, the condition is often treatable and reversible.

Speech disorders. Many post-stroke victims suffer speech disorders, and in some cases other neurological problems cause these disorders.

Headache. The most common neurological complaint. Most go away with aspirin or other painkillers. Some, such as migraines, can be complex and require specialized treatment. Some neurologists have a special interest in complex headache problems.

Peripheral nerve disorders. This includes injuries or disorders to the nervous system other than the brain or spinal cord, such as to the extremities.

Cancer. A rare special interest. This area concentrates on cancer of the nervous system and chemotherapies more effective in neurologic cancer. More properly called neuro-oncology.

Neurologic eye disorders. The specialists in this field appear under a subsection of eye specialists called neuro-ophthalmology.

Pediatric. Pediatric neurologists appear under pediatric neurology. In some cases, individuals are known for their work in both pediatric and adult neurology and are listed in both sections.

The vast majority of neurologists listed here practice general neurology but have special interests in some neurological problems. The majority of them treat the full range of neurologic disorders. Some, however, have narrowed their scope to one or two types of problems. The vast majority of them are also located at centers where a variety of specialized care is available.

NEUROLOGISTS

Dr. Raymond D. Adams
Massachusetts General Hospital
Boston, Massachusetts 02114

Chairman emeritus, department of neurology.

Dr. Alberto Aguayo
(peripheral nerve disorders)
Montreal General Hospital
Montreal, Quebec
Canada H3G 1A4

Dr. J. Norman Allen (cancer)
University Hospital
466 West Tenth Avenue
Columbus, Ohio 43210

Professor and director of the division of neurology.

Dr. Stanley Appel
Baylor College of Medicine
Houston, Texas 77030

Professor and chairman, department of neurology.

Dr. Arthur Asbury (peripheral nerve disorders)
Hospital of the University of Pennsylvania
Philadelphia, Pennsylvania 19104

Professor and chairman, department of neurology.

Dr. A. B. Baker
Mt. Sinai Hospital
2215 Park Avenue South
Minneapolis, Minnesota 55404

Professor emeritus of neurology, Minnesota.

Dr. Leonard Berg
4989 Barnes Hospital Plaza
St. Louis, Missouri 63110

Professor of clinical neurology, Washington University.

Dr. Walter Bradley
(neuromuscular diseases)
Tufts University Medical School
Boston, Massachusetts 02111

Professor of neurology.

Dr. Michael Brooke
(neuromuscular diseases)
Department of Neurology
Washington University Medical School
49 Barnes Hospital Plaza
St. Louis, Missouri 63110

Professor of neurology.

Dr. Roger Broughton (epilepsy)
Department of Medicine
Ottawa General Hospital
43 Bruyere
Ottawa, Ontario
Canada K1N 5C8

Dr. John Calverly
University of Texas Medical Branch
Galveston, Texas 77550

Professor and chairman, department of neurology.

Dr. Kenneth L. Casey (pain)
University of Michigan Medical Center
Ann Arbor, Michigan 48109

Professor of physiology and associate professor of neurology.

Dr. Donald Dalessio (headache)
Scripps Clinic
La Jolla, California 92037

Dr. Daniel B. Drachman
(neuromuscular diseases)
The Johns Hopkins Medical School
Baltimore, Maryland 21205

Professor of neurology.

Dr. Peter J. Dyck
(peripheral nerve diseases)
Mayo Clinic
Rochester, Minnesota 55901

Dr. Andrew G. Engel
(neuromuscular diseases)
Mayo Clinic
Rochester, Minnesota 55901

Dr. C. Miller Fisher
(cerebrovascular diseases)
Massachusetts General Hospital
Boston, Massachusetts 02114

Dr. Robert Fishman
University of California Medical Center
San Francisco, California 94143

Professor and chairman, department of neurology.

Dr. Arnold Friedman (headache)
The Neurological Institute
710 West 168th Street
New York, New York 10032

Dr. Norman Geschwind
(speech disorders)
Beth Israel Hospital
Boston, Massachusetts 02215

Professor of neurology, Harvard.

Dr. Gilbert H. Glaser (epilepsy)
Yale University Medical School
New Haven, Connecticut 06510

Professor of neurology.

Dr. Norman Goldstein
Mayo Clinic
Rochester, Minnesota 55901

Professor of neurology, Mayo.

Dr. James F. Hammill
Neurological Institute
710 West 168th Street
New York, New York 10032

Associate professor of neurology, Columbia.

Dr. Robert Herndon
(multiple sclerosis)
Center for Brain Research
University of Rochester
Rochester, New York 14642

Professor of neurology.

Dr. T. R. Johns (myasthenia gravis)
University of Virginia Medical Center
Charlottesville, Virginia 22901

Professor of neurology.

Dr. Richard Johnson
(viral diseases, multiple sclerosis)
Johns Hopkins Medical School
Baltimore, Maryland 21205

*Eisenhower professor of neurology
and microbiology.*

Dr. Robert J. Joynt
Center for Brain Research
University of Rochester
Rochester, New York 14642

*Professor and chairman, department
of neurology.*

Dr. George Kapatti
(neuromuscular diseases)
The Montreal Neurologic Institute
Montreal, Quebec
Canada H3A 2D4

Dr. Herbert R. Karp
Emory University Hospital
Atlanta, Georgia 30303

*Chief of neurology section;
professor and chairman, department
of neurology.*

Dr. William M. Landau
(movement disorders)
Washington University Medical
School
St. Louis, Missouri 63110

Professor of neurology.

Dr. Irwin Levy
4989 Barnes Hospital Plaza
St. Louis, Missouri 63110

*Professor of clinical neurology,
Washington University*

Dr. Guy M. McKhann
Department of Neurology
The Johns Hopkins Medical School
Baltimore, Maryland 21205

Kennedy professor of neurology.

Dr. Michael P. McQuillen
(neuromuscular diseases)
Medical College of Wisconsin
Milwaukee, Wisconsin 53226

*Professor and chairman, department
of neurology.*

Dr. Oscar Marin (speech and
learning disorders)
The Johns Hopkins Medical School
Baltimore, Maryland 21205

Professor of neurology.

Dr. Joseph Martin
(neuroendocrinology)
Massachusetts General Hospital
Boston, Massachusetts 02114

*Chairman, department of neurology,
Harvard. Neuroendocrinology
involves disorders of endocrine
glands caused by neurology
problems.*

Dr. Jerry R. Mendell
(neuromuscular diseases)
University Hospital
466 West Tenth Street
Columbus, Ohio 43210

*Associate professor of neurology,
Ohio State.*

Dr. Clark Millikan
(cerebrovascular diseases)
University of Utah Medical School
Salt Lake City, Utah 84132

Professor of neurology.

Dr. Jay P. Mohr
(speech disorders)
Department of Neurology
University of South Alabama
Medical School
Mobile, Alabama 36617

*Professor and chairman, department
of neurology.*

Dr. Donald W. Mulder
Mayo Clinic
Rochester, Minnesota 55901

Dr. Theodore Munsat
(neuromuscular disorders)
Tufts University Medical School
Boston, Massachusetts 02111

Professor of neurology.

Dr. Audrey S. Penn
Neurological Institute
710 West 168th Street
New York, New York 10032

Associate professor of neurology.

Dr. Fred Plum
New York Hospital–Cornell
Medical Center
525 East 68th Street
New York, New York 10021

Anne Parrish Titzell professor and chairman, department of neurology, Cornell.

Dr. Jerome Posner (cancer)
Memorial Hospital for Cancer and
Allied Diseases
1275 York Avenue
New York, New York 10021

Professor of neurology, Cornell.

Dr. Oscar Reinmuth
University of Pittsburgh Medical
School
Pittsburgh, Pennsylvania 15213

Professor of neurology.

Dr. Roger N. Rosenberg
Department of Neurology
Southwestern Medical School
Dallas, Texas 75235

Professor and chairman, department of neurology.

Dr. Lewis P. Rowland
(neuromuscular diseases)
Neurological Institute
710 West 168th Street
New York, New York 10032

Dr. Herbert H. Schaumburg
(neurotoxicology)
Albert Einstein Medical School
1300 Morris Park Avenue
Bronx, New York 10461

*Professor of neurology.
Neurotoxicology deals with
the effects of poisons on the
nervous system.*

Dr. Peritz Scheinberg
(cerebrovascular diseases)
Department of Neurology
University of Miami Medical School
Biscayne Annex
Miami, Florida 33152

*Professor and chairman, department
of neurology.*

Dr. Stuart Schneck
University of Colorado Medical
School
Denver, Colorado 80262

Professor of neurology.

Dr. Donald L. Schotland
(neuromuscular diseases)
Hospital of the University of
Pennsylvania
Philadelphia, Pennsylvania 19104

*Professor of neurology; director,
Watts Neuromuscular Research
Center.*

Dr. Donald H. Silberberg
(multiple sclerosis)
Hospital of the University of
Pennsylvania
Philadelphia, Pennsylvania 19104

Professor of neurology.

Dr. Philip D. Swanson
Department of Neurology
University of Washington Medical School
Seattle, Washington 98195

Professor of neurology.

Dr. James Toole
(cerebrovascular diseases)
Bowman-Grey Medical School
Winston-Salem, North Carolina 27109

Professor and chairman, department of neurology.

Dr. H. Richard Tyler
Peter Bent Brigham Hospital
Boston, Massachusetts 02115

Professor of neurology, Harvard.

Dr. Maurice Van Allen
University Hospitals
Iowa City, Iowa 52242

Professor of neurology.

Dr. Nicholas A. Vick (cancer)
2650 Ridge Avenue
Evanston, Illinois 60201

Professor of neurology, Northwestern University Medical School.

Dr. Leslie P. Weiner (viral diseases)
University of Southern California
School of Medicine
McKibben 142
2025 Zonal Avenue
Los Angeles, California 90033

Professor of neurology and microbiology.

Dr. Jack P. Whisnant
(cerebrovascular diseases)
Mayo Clinic
Rochester, Minnesota 55901

Professor and chairman, department of neurology, Mayo.

Dr. John Whitaker
(multiple sclerosis)
University of Tennessee Medical Center
Memphis, Tennessee 38163

Chiefly a researcher, but sees some patients.

Dr. Melvin D. Yahr
(movement disorders)
Mt. Sinai Hospital
100th Street and Fifth Avenue
New York, New York 10029

Dr. Frank Yatsu
(cerebrovascular diseases)
University of Oregon Center
for Health Sciences
Portland, Oregon 97201

Professor and chairman, department of neurology.

Dr. Dewey K. Zeigler (headache)
University of Kansas Medical Center
Kansas City, Kansas 66103

Professor of neurology.

Neurosurgeons

Neurosurgery is the most technically demanding of all surgical disciplines. It requires the utmost precision and expertise to get the best possible results for the patient. The most significant breakthrough in neurosurgery in recent years is the development of the operating microscope. This microscope, which requires special training to learn to use under surgical conditions, enlarges the field of view of the neurosurgeon some 15 times and greatly intensifies the light. "It allows us to preserve and protect small vessels and to get an enormously better look at the area in which we are operating," one neurosurgeon said.

The microscope has virtually revolutionized both pituitary gland and aneurysm surgery, both very difficult neurological procedures. What can the microscope mean in terms of results for the patient? If you have an aneurysm (a potentially life-threatening enlargement of a weakened blood vessel in the brain), you have only a 50 percent chance of returning to normal if you are operated on by a neurosurgeon who is not trained to operate the neurosurgical microscope. However, if you are operated on by a skilled neurosurgeon who is trained to use the microscope (everyone on this list is expertly trained in its use), your chance of leaving the hospital in a back-to-normal condition is increased to about 90 percent. Fortunately, the majority of the 3,000 neurosurgeons operating in this country today use the operating microscope, and the survival and recovery rates for many neurologic procedures have increased.

Unlike many other medical specialties, neurosurgeons are generally considered to be at their peak at a younger age. Some neurosurgeons consider the peak years to be from the late thirties to the mid-fifties. Others feel, however, that many neurosurgeons operate with as much skill and better judgment well into their sixties. One reason for the emphasis on youth is not just the dexterity and steadiness that youth usually provides, but because the enormous emotional strain neurosurgery places on doctors takes its toll. "There is a lot of grief in neurosurgery and you have to be able to stand up to that," one experienced neurosurgeon said. "It can be very draining over a long period of time." Another neurosurgeon remarked: "Your fatigue factor increases as you get older and the long procedures are tiring, but also your judgment is better. If you could find where these two processes intersect, where your stamina is still superb and your judgment refined, you would have the perfect age for a neurosurgeon. I suspect it varies from one neurosurgeon to another."

One problem with neurosurgery today is that there are more neurosurgeons operating than there are patients in real need of neurosurgery. This causes two problems: The first is that the average neurosurgeon does not get to see very many unusual cases and therefore when he is presented with one he often does not have an adequate backlog of experience to know how best to deal with it. The second result of our overabundance of neurosurgeons is that there may be too many unnecessary neurosurgical procedures, most specifically disc operations. The disc procedure, which can be performed adequately by any good neurosurgeon, is often performed when other, less invasive therapies might be as successful, according to many neurosurgeons.

Unlike some of the other surgical specialties, such as heart surgery and kidney transplants, there is no audit or statistical evaluation by which to compare the success or failure of various neurosurgeons or neurological institutions. However, as one neurosurgeon noted, "There are a few areas in which surgery should be performed only by a very few neurosurgeons. In these specific areas the difference in the results to the patient is very spectacular."

Although most neurosurgeons operate on a wide range of neurological problems, some of them tend to subspecialize in specific areas. The generally recognized subspecialties of adult neurosurgery are:

1. *Cerebrovascular surgery.* This generally concerns itself with aneurysm and vascular by-pass surgery and arterial surgery in the neck.

2. *Brain tumor surgery.* Malignant brain tumors do not have a much better prognosis than they did ten or twenty years ago because it is difficult to get all the malignancy out of the brain tissue without inflicting grave neurological damage on the patient. However, fewer than half of all brain tumors are malignant. Paradoxically, nonmalignant tumors often prove more difficult to remove than malignant ones.

3. *Pain surgery.* Facial pain, once intractable, can now be alleviated or stopped entirely by a relatively new surgical technique. Other forms

of neurological and cancer pain can also be ended through surgical techniques.

4. *Pituitary gland surgery.* The pituitary gland is located in the brain and is the master endocrine gland for the human body. Like aneurysm surgery, perhaps the greatest strides in neurosurgery have been made in this area because of the operating microscope. The most common pituitary procedure is for removal of a tumor, or for removing the stimulating effect of the growth of other tumors, such as breast tumors.

5. *Trauma.* A frequent result of neurological trauma is a blood clot on the brain or damage to the spinal cord or peripheral nervous system.

6. *Seizure surgery.* For epilepsy, a convulsive disorder, this is a rarer form of neurological surgery. It is a last resort when drugs and other medical means fail to stop seizures.

7. *Disc surgery.* This is the bread and butter of neurosurgeons, and except in unusual cases, a procedure any board certified neurosurgeon should be able to perform adequately. However, some neurosurgeons have specific interests in the more difficult or unusual disc problems.

8. *Acoustic or ear-related tumors.* This is an area of overlap between neurosurgeons and otolaryngologists (ear, nose, and throat surgeons). Specialists in both areas perform it, but neurosurgeons generally do acoustic tumor surgery when the tumors are larger and cannot be removed through the ear or when they are within the cranium.

9. *Peripheral nerve surgery.* This involves parts of the nervous system outside of the brain. Surgery usually involves tumors or injury repair.

10. *Stereotactic surgery.* Also called physiologic surgery, this involves deep needle probes into the brain using x-ray for guidance. This type of surgery is for the relief of pain and, in rare cases, also for Parkinson's disease and for other motor disorders that do not respond to drug therapy.

These ten special interest areas are not all recognized subspecialties of neurosurgery. Only *cerebrovascular surgery, stereotactic surgery,* and *pediatric neurological surgery* are recognized subspecialties. Although some of the neurologic surgeons listed here do pediatric work, specialized pediatric neurosurgeons are listed separately in the pediatric section. It should also be emphasized that most neurosurgeons perform the full range of neurological surgery from aneurysms to tumors, but some tend to concentrate in the areas designated.

NEUROSURGEONS

Dr. Shelly Chou
Department of Neurologic Surgery
University of Minnesota
Minneapolis, Minnesota 55404
Professor and chairman, department of neurosurgery.

Dr. W. Kemp Clark
University of Texas, Southwestern
Medical School
5323 Harry Hines Boulevard
Dallas, Texas 75235
Professor and chairman, division of neurosurgery.

Dr. William Collins (pituitary tumors and spinal injury)
Yale University Medical School
333 Cedar Street
New Haven, Connecticut 06510
Professor of neurosurgery.

Dr. Donald F. Dohn
Cleveland Clinic
9500 Euclid Avenue
Cleveland, Ohio 44106
Chief of neurosurgery.

Dr. Charles G. Drake
(cerebrovascular surgery)
Dr. Sidney Peerless
339 Windemere Road
University Hospital
London, Ontario
Canada
Dr. Drake is the most experienced aneurysm surgeon in the world and has handled the most difficult cases. Dr. Peerless is his younger associate who is assuming more of the surgical duties and has succeeded Dr. Drake as chief of neurosurgery. Dr. Drake is chief of surgery.

Dr. William H. Feindel
(seizure surgery)
Montreal Neurological Institute
3801 University Street
Montreal, Quebec
Canada H3A 2D4
The Montreal Neurologic Institute is known internationally for seizure surgery.

Dr. Sidney Goldring
(seizure surgery)
Barnes Hospital Plaza
St. Louis, Missouri 63110
Professor and head of neurosurgery, Washington University.

Dr. Jules Hardy
(pituitary surgery)
Montreal Neurological Institute
3801 University Street
Montreal, Quebec
Canada H3A 2D4

Dr. Julian T. Hoff (head injury)
Department of Neurosurgery
University of California Medical Center
San Francisco, California 94143
Associate professor of neurosurgery.

Dr. William E. Hunt
(cerebrovascular surgery)
410 West Tenth Avenue
Columbus, Ohio 43210
Professor and director, division of neurologic surgery, Ohio State University College of Medicine.

Dr. Peter J. Jannetta
(pain relief and facial spasms)
Presbyterian-University Hospital
230 Lothrop Street
Pittsburgh, Pennsylvania 15213

Professor and chairman, department of neurosurgery, University of Pittsburgh Medical School.

Dr. Robert B. King
750 East Adams Street
Syracuse, New York 13210

Professor and chairman, department of neurosurgery, State University of New York.

Dr. David G. Kline
(peripheral nerve surgery)
Louisiana State University Medical School
1542 Tulane Avenue
New Orleans, Louisiana 70112

Professor of surgery (neurosurgery).

Dr. Theodore Kurze (microsurgery)
111 Congress Street B
Pasadena, California 91105

Professor and chairman, department of neurosurgery, University of Southern California.

Dr. Edward R. Laws, Jr.
(pituitary and brain tumor)
Mayo Clinic
Rochester, Minnesota 55901

Dr. Donlin M. Long (pain)
The Johns Hopkins Hospital
Baltimore, Maryland 21205

Professor and director, department of neurosurgery.

Dr. Stephen Mahaley (brain tumors)
University of North Carolina
Chapel Hill, North Carolina 27514

Chief, division of neurosurgery.

Dr. Leonard I. Malis (microsurgery)
1176 Fifth Avenue
New York, New York 10029

Professor and director, department of neurosurgery, Mt. Sinai School of Medicine.

Dr. Joseph C. Maroon
University of Pittsburgh
Pittsburgh, Pennsylvania 15261

Associate professor of neurosurgery.

Dr. Jost Michelson
Columbia-Presbyterian Hospital
710 West 168th Street
New York, New York 10032

Associate professor of neurosurgery at Columbia.

Dr. Ross H. Miller
Mayo Clinic
Rochester, Minnesota 55901

Chief of neurosurgery at Mayo.

Dr. J. F. Mullan (stereotactic pain surgery)
University of Chicago Hospital
950 East 59th Street
Chicago, Illinois 60637

Chief of neurosurgery.

Dr. George A. Ojemann
(seizure surgery)
University of Washington Medical School
Seattle, Washington 98195

Associate professor of neurosurgery.

Dr. Robert G. Ojemann
(cerebrovascular surgery and acoustic tumors)
Massachusetts General Hospital
Boston, Massachusetts 02114

Associate clinical professor of surgery, Harvard.

Dr. Russell H. Patterson, Jr.
New York Hospital
525 East 68th Street
New York, New York 10021

Professor of surgery and neurosurgery, Cornell Medical School.

Dr. Robert Rand
(microsurgery)
University of California at Los Angeles Medical Center
Los Angeles, California 90024

Professor of neurosurgery.

Dr. Joseph Ransohoff
(cerebrovascular and tumor surgery)
New York University Medical School
550 First Avenue
New York, New York 10016

Chairman, department of neurosurgery.

Dr. Albert L. Rhoton, Jr.
(microsurgery and acoustic tumors)
University of Florida
Gainesville, Florida 32601

Professor and chairman, department of neurosurgery. Leader in microsurgical techniques and teaching. Also known for facial pain surgery.

Dr. Hugo Rizzoli
2150 Pennsylvania Avenue, NW
Washington, District of Columbia 20037

Professor and chairman, department of neurosurgery, George Washington University Medical School.

Dr. James T. Robertson
(vascular and brain tumor)
920 Madison
Memphis, Tennessee 38103

Professor and chairman, department of neurosurgery, University of Tennessee.

Dr. Robert G. Selker (brain tumor)
University of Pittsburgh
Pittsburgh, Pennsylvania 15261

Professor of neurosurgery.

Dr. Frederick A. Simeone
(unusual back and disc problems)
Hospital of the University of Pennsylvania
3400 Spruce Street
Philadelphia, Pennsylvania 19104

Associate professor of neurosurgery, University of Pennsylvania Medical School.

Dr. W. Eugene Stern
University of California at Los Angeles Medical Center
Los Angeles, California 90024

Professor and chairman, department of surgery and neurosurgery.

Dr. Thoralf Sundt (cerebrovascular)
Mayo Clinic
Rochester, Minnesota 55901

Dr. John M. Tew, Jr. (vascular and stereotactic facial pain surgery)
Mayfield Neurological Institute
506 Oak Street
Cincinnati, Ohio 45219

Director of neurosurgical services, Good Samaritan and Deaconess hospitals.

Dr. George T. Tindall
(pituitary surgery)
Emory University Hospital
1365 Clifton Road, NE
Atlanta, Georgia 30322

*Professor of surgery; chief,
division of neurosurgery.*

Dr. Robert H. Wilkins
Duke Medical Center
Durham, North Carolina 27710

*Professor and chairman, division of
neurosurgery.*

Dr. Charles B. Wilson
(brain tumor surgery)
University of California Medical
Center
San Francisco, California 94143

*Professor and chairman, department
of neurosurgery.*

Dr. Nicholas T. Zervas
(pituitary surgery)
Massachusetts General Hospital
Boston, Massachusetts 02114

*Professor of neurosurgery, Harvard;
chief of neurosurgical services,
Massachusetts General.*

Depression

Depression is the most common mental illness, and the most treatable. All of us during some time in our life have felt depressed. However, clinical depression—that is, a depression which can be diagnosed under clinical circumstances—is a very different disorder from feeling the blues.

The term depression covers a wide spectrum of disorders. At one end are the relatively milder depressions, usually secondary to an event, such as the death of a husband or wife or parent, or a divorce or loss of a job. Although painful, they do not often result in major problems of functioning. This type of depression involves some biochemical predisposition in origin, which nevertheless may have been triggered by a grief reaction to an event. At the other end of the spectrum is major depression, which involves more complex and more debilitating symptoms. The causes of major depression are likely to involve both your genes and your situation in life.

Major depression can be either unipolar (depression only) or bipolar, in which the patient experiences both depressive and manic episodes. Unlike unipolar depression, bipolar depression is characterized by wild swings in mood—from ecstasy to despair.

Some depressive episodes are psychotic in nature and include hallucinations, delusions, and paranoia. Also, the sense of pain and despair a truly depressed person feels is unimaginable to those of us who have only suffered the blues.

How is depression treated? Historically, there has been a split in psychiatry between those who believed depression was only biochemical in nature and those who believed it was only psychological. This split is diminishing now and, as one psychiatrist says, "I don't think you can find many psychiatrists who would think there is no biological basis to major depression." He also noted, "I think depression treatment should be thought of as two things; one, treat the illness with drugs, and two, treat the person with psychotherapy. Both are needed for successful treatment."

This psychiatrist, who represents a blend of the two schools, suggests that the best approach to depression treatment involves both psychotherapy and drug therapy because of the interrelationship of the causes of depression. He also suggests that psychiatrists more recently trained are more likely to offer a better balance than those trained earlier.

What are the signs of major depression and how do they differ from less severe depressions or from an ordinary case of the blues? Here are a few of the generally recognized signs:

1. *Persistent feelings of hopelessness, sadness, and depression.* These feelings persist for more than two weeks.

2. *Sleep disturbances.* Either excessive sleepiness or, more likely, inability to sleep well, including awakening at night or early in the morning.

3. *Appetite disturbances.* Either eating too little or too much, but usually involves a loss of appetite.

4. *Noticeable loss of energy.* A general listlessness even in activities you formerly enjoyed.

5. *A decreased ability to concentrate.*

6. *Generally slowed thinking.* A loss of alertness and responsiveness.

7. *Feelings of guilt or blame.*

8. *Recurrent thoughts of suicide or death.*

Not all of these symptoms need appear, but, coupled with a general feeling of hopelessness, if *five* of them do appear and continue for at least two weeks, you may well be clinically depressed and in need of therapy.

While these symptoms seem straightforward, it should be emphasized that depression can be misdiagnosed by unskilled psychiatrists. Some of its symptoms can be mistaken for other mental disorders. Says one prominent psychiatrist: "The best clinicians can both diagnose the illness properly and then treat it properly. If it doesn't respond well to certain drugs, the skilled psychiatrist knows when to change them and what to give the patient next. He knows the full range of drugs and he knows how the patient should be approached for psychotherapy. At the major centers, we see patients on whom other psychiatrists have given up because they are stuck."

Below are listed some of the leading psychiatrists noted for their understanding and treatment of depression. The amount of patient care they handle varies, but they and their units do handle the difficult cases of depression.

PSYCHIATRISTS SPECIALIZING IN DEPRESSION

Dr. Aaron T. Beck
University of Pennsylvania
133 South 36th Street
Philadelphia, Pennsylvania 19104

Professor of psychiatry. Dr. Beck is known for his cognitive therapy approach to depression in which the patient is shown that his low self-esteem is an incorrect self-image.

Dr. Bernard Carroll
Mental Health Research Unit
University of Michigan
Medical School
Ann Arbor, Michigan 48104

Dr. Carroll is professor of psychiatry and director of the Mental Health Research Unit.

Dr. Paula Clayton
Department of Psychiatry
Washington University
Medical School
St. Louis, Missouri 63110

Dr. John M. Davis
Illinois State Psychiatric Unit
1601 West Taylor Street
Chicago, Illinois 60620

Professor of psychiatry at the University of Chicago; director of research at the Psychiatric Unit.

Dr. Ronald R. Fieve
New York State Psychiatric Institute
722 West 168th Street
New York, New York 10032

Professor of clinical psychiatry at Columbia College of Physicians and Surgeons. Dr. Fieve is known as a leading expert in the treatment of manic depression with lithium.

Dr. Frederick Goodwin
Clinical Center, Intra-mural
Research Program
National Institute of Mental Health
Bethesda, Maryland 20014

As in all National Institutes of Health clinical care programs, there is no charge. However, patients require referrals from other physicians and must meet National Institutes of Health research protocols. In addition to his National Institutes of Health work, Dr. Goodwin does see private patients, and is especially interested in the interrelationships between drugs and psychotherapy.

Dr. David S. Janowsky
University Hospital
Department of Psychiatry
225 West Dickinson
San Diego, California 92103

Professor of psychiatry, University of California at San Diego. Director of psychiatric services at University Hospital.

Dr. Donald Klein
New York State Psychiatric Institute
722 West 168th Street
New York, New York 10032

Professor of psychiatry at Columbia. Director of psychiatric research at the New York State Psychiatric Institute.

Dr. Nathan S. Kline
130 East 77th Street
New York, New York 10021

Dr. Kline is in private practice.

Dr. James W. Maas
Department of Psychiatry
Yale University Medical School
333 Cedar Street
New Haven, Connecticut 06510

Professor of psychiatry at Yale.

Dr. Myer Mendleson
The Institute of the Pennsylvania Hospital
111 North 49th Street
Philadelphia, Pennsylvania 19139

Professor of clinical psychiatry, University of Pennsylvania; senior attending psychiatrist, the Institute of the Pennsylvania Hospital.

Dr. Arthur J. Prange, Jr.
Department of Psychiatry
University of North Carolina
Medical School
Chapel Hill, North Carolina 27514

Professor and director of research, University of North Carolina Medical School.

Dr. R. Bruce Sloan
Los Angeles County–University of Southern California Medical Center
1200 North State Street
Los Angeles, California 90033

Professor and chairman, department of psychiatry.

Dr. Eberhardt Ulenhuth
Department of Psychiatry
University of Chicago
Medical School
950 East 59th Street
Chicago, Illinois 60637

Professor of psychiatry.

Myrna Weissman, Ph.D.
Connecticut Mental Health Center
Depression Research Center
904 Howard Avenue
New Haven, Connecticut 06519

A heavy emphasis on research but the center does see many patients. Affiliated with Yale University.

Dr. George Winokur
Department of Psychiatry
University of Iowa Medical School
Iowa City, Iowa 52240

Chairman of the psychiatry department at Iowa.

Diseases of the Eye

❧ ➤➤➤✕⳹⳹⳹ ❧

Subspecialties of Ophthalmology

Because of the complexity and precision required in most eye surgery, ophthalmologists generally subspecialize in different diseases or in different parts of the eye. This is particularly true for the most complicated diseases and surgery involving difficult procedures. Routine procedures such as uncomplicated cataract removal and evaluations for disease or glasses can be done by any board certified ophthalmologist. The following are the basic subspecialties of ophthalmology and the areas in which the skill and experience of the physician can make an enormous difference in the result to the patient.

Glaucoma. Glaucoma is a disease which causes the loss of eyesight because of increased pressure within the eye. Although it remains one of the leading causes of blindness and visual disability, in most cases if it is diagnosed early (a simple procedure) it can be treated by medication and damage can be prevented. In cases of more severe glaucoma uncontrolled by medicine, surgery can often prevent damage or cure the disease. In some types of glaucoma, a laser beam can be of help in treatment and in preventing the need for surgery.

Cornea and external disease. The cornea is the transparent membrane at the front of the eye which helps bend and focus light rays. Corneal infections caused by virus, bacteria, fungus, allergic reaction, and other conditions, such as edema of the cornea, keratoconus (thinning of the cornea), or trauma, can cause serious visual loss, or blindness, and can be painful. In cases of permanent cornea damage from these or other causes—including chemicals—a corneal transplant can restore sight. In the most suitable cases of blindness, corneal transplants have a 90 percent success rate. In cases of chemical blinding, however, the success rate is considerably lower.

Retina. Diabetic retinopathy, in which diabetes damages the retina and causes visual loss and blindness, is a frequent complication of diabetes and a leading cause of blindness. Also, retina detachment, from injury or other causes, is another hazard to the retina. The vitreous (the clear gel that fills the center of the eye) can also be damaged secondarily by diabetic retinopathy, and this too can cause severe vision loss. While these are bleak complications, remarkable progress has been made in retina and vitreous surgery. A national clinical study sponsored by the National Institutes of Health has shown conclusively that a procedure called *photocoagulation* (using argon laser or xenon arc beams) can successfully seal off or destroy abnormal retinal blood vessels and can prevent hemorrhaging in the eye. A surgical procedure called vitrectomy may achieve some restoration of sight if the vitreous has been damaged. Many people who have had vitrectomies have had their sight restored; some have had it restored well enough to read.

Neuro-ophthalmology. Neuro-ophthalmology is a subspecialty which deals with visual and eye movement problems that involve the nervous system or are due to a nervous system disorder. Both neurologists and ophthalmologists have a special interest in this area, and outstanding specialists from both fields are listed here. The symptoms of a neuro-ophthalmological disorder can be sudden blindness, eye movement disorders, headaches, double vision, half field vision (in which only half of an object is seen), and swollen nerve heads in the back of the eye which may not cause any symptoms but which can be detected in a routine eye exam.

Ophthalmic-Plastic Surgery. This is a relatively smaller and newer subspecialty which involves surgery to correct problems in the eye orbit, the eyelids, and the tearing (or lachrymal) system. These problems can include serious eye injury, congenital malformations, scarring, and tumors. Perhaps the most common ophthalmic-plastic referrals are for surgery to correct excessive eye tearing caused by tear duct obstruction, or surgery to correct excessively heavy eyelids which can adversely affect appearance and sight. Also, tumors in the orbit, either in the bony or the fleshy part, and eyelid tumors are special interests of ophthalmic-plastic surgeons. Also, as the name of the subspecialty suggests, the techniques of plastic surgery are involved, particularly in cosmetic work to improve the eye's appearance. Some plastic surgeons also do reconstructive work in the area of the eye.

Pediatric. Pediatric eye specialists are listed in the pediatric section.

GLAUCOMA SPECIALISTS

Dr. Douglas R. Anderson
Bascom-Palmer Eye Institute
University of Miami Medical School
1638 NW Tenth Avenue
Miami, Florida 33136

*Associate professor of
ophthalmology.*

Dr. Mansour F. Armaly
George Washington
University Hospital
2150 Pennsylvania Avenue, NW
Washington, District of Columbia
20037

*Professor and chairman, department
of ophthalmology.*

Dr. Richard Brubaker
Mayo Clinic
Rochester, Minnesota 55901

Dr. Max Forbes
Columbia-Presbyterian
Medical Center
635 West 165th Street
New York, New York 10032

*Associate professor of
ophthalmology.*

Dr. Joseph S. Haas
1725 West Harrison Street
Chicago, Illinois 60612

*Professor of ophthalmology,
Rush Medical College.*

Dr. Thomas B. Hutchinson
10 Hawthorne Place
Boston, Massachusetts 02114

*Assistant clinical professor
of ophthalmology, Harvard.*

Dr. Allen K. Kolker
Washington University
Medical School
4901 Barnes Hospital Plaza
St. Louis, Missouri 63110

Professor of ophthalmology.

Dr. Paul Lichter
University of Michigan
Medical Center
Ann Arbor, Michigan 48109

*Professor and chairman, department
of ophthalmology.*

Dr. Charles D. Phelps
University Hospitals
Iowa City, Iowa 52242

*Assistant professor of
ophthalmology, University of Iowa
Medical School.*

Dr. Robert N. Shaffer
490 Post Street
San Francisco, California 94132

*Clinical professor of ophthalmology,
University of California.
Associates Dunbar Hoskins and
Jack Heatherington are also
considered outstanding.*

Dr. Richard Simmons
100 Charles River Plaza–
Cambridge Street
Boston, Massachusetts 02114

Assistant clinical professor of ophthalmology, Harvard; surgeon, Massachusetts Eye and Ear Infirmary.

Dr. George L. Spaeth
Wills Eye Hospital
1601 Spring Garden Street
Philadelphia, Pennsylvania 19103

Director of glaucoma service.

CORNEA AND EXTERNAL EYE DISEASE SPECIALISTS

(As mentioned earlier, some cornea specialists have a special interest in corneal infections. They are so noted.)

Dr. Jules L. Baum
Tufts–New England Medical Center
171 Harrison Street
Boston, Massachusetts 02111

A special interest in infections. Professor of ophthalmology.

Dr. S. Arthur Boruchoff
100 Charles River Plaza
Boston, Massachusetts 02114

Associate clinical professor of ophthalmology, Harvard.

Dr. Stuart Brown
The Eye and Ear Hospital
230 Lothrup Street
Pittsburgh, Pennsylvania 15213

Professor and chairman, department of ophthalmology, University of Pittsburgh.

Dr. Jorge N. Buxton
New York Eye and Ear Infirmary
310 East 14th Street
New York, New York 10003

Clinical associate professor of medicine, New Jersey College of Medicine.

Dr. H. Dwight Cavanagh
Emory University Hospital
Atlanta, Georgia 30322

Professor and chairman, department of ophthalmology. A special interest in infections.

Dr. John W. Chandler
Ophthalmic Consultants Northwest
700 Broadway
Seattle, Washington 98122

Dr. Claes H. Dohlman
Massachusetts Eye and Ear
Infirmary
243 Charles Street
Boston, Massachusetts 02114

Chief of eye service; professor and chairman of ophthalmology, Harvard.

Dr. Max Fine
2233 Post Street
San Francisco, California 94115

Clinical professor of ophthalmology, University of California.

Dr. Richard K. Forster
Bascom-Palmer Eye Institute
University of Miami Medical School
1638 NW Tenth Avenue
Miami, Florida 33136

*Assistant professor of
ophthalmology. A special interest
in external eye infections.*

Dr. Dan B. Jones
Baylor College of Medicine
Houston, Texas 77025

*Known for his work on infectious
external eye diseases.*

Dr. Herbert Kaufman
Louisiana State University Eye
Center
136 South Ronan Street
New Orleans, Louisiana 70116

*Professor of ophthalmology and
pharmacology; director, Louisiana
State University Eye Center. Also
known for his interest in external
viral eye infections.*

Dr. Peter Laibson
Wills Eye Hospital
1601 Spring Garden Street
Philadelphia, Pennsylvania 19130

*Professor of ophthalmology,
Jefferson Medical College.*

Dr. Michael Lemp
Foxhall Square
3301 New Mexico Avenue, NW
Washington, District of Columbia
20016

*Director of corneal services,
Georgetown University Hospital.*

Dr. Anthony Nesburn
620 South San Vicente Boulevard
Los Angeles, California 90048

*Head of Corneal Clinic and Eye
Bank, Los Angeles County–
University of Southern California
Medical Center.*

Dr. David Paton
The Cullen Eye Institute
Baylor College of Medicine
Houston, Texas 77030

*Professor and chairman, department
of ophthalmology.*

Dr. Thomas H. Pettit
Jules Stein Eye Institute
University of California at Los
Angeles Medical Center
Los Angeles, California 90024

*Professor of ophthalmology;
director of Cornea-External Ocular
Disease Service.*

Dr. Roswell Pfister
1720 Eighth Avenue
Birmingham, Alabama 35233

*Professor and chairman, combined
program in ophthalmology,
University of Alabama.*

Dr. Walter Stark
Wilmer Eye Institute
The Johns Hopkins Hospital
Baltimore, Maryland 21205

Dr. Richard Troutman
755 Park Avenue
New York, New York 10021

*Professor and chairman, department
of ophthalmology, State University
of New York Downstate
(Brooklyn).*

SPECIALISTS IN RETINAL AND VITREOUS DISEASES

(Although virtually every retina specialist performs vitreous surgery, some are noted for their special interest in vitreous surgery and are so noted.)

Dr. Thomas M. Aaberg
Wisconsin Medical College
Milwaukee, Wisconsin 53226

Associate professor of ophthalmology.

Dr. Lloyd H. Aiello
William Beethan Eye Unit
Joslin Clinic
1 Joslin Place
Boston, Massachusetts 02215

Known especially for his work with diabetic eye problems.

Dr. Morton S. Cox
Parkview Medical Building
100 Wall Street
Ann Arbor, Michigan 48109

Director of retina services at University of Michigan Medical Center.

Dr. Mathew D. Davis
Eye Clinic
University of Wisconsin Medical School
Madison, Wisconsin 53706

Professor of ophthalmology, known for his work in diabetic retinopathy.

Dr. J. Graham Dobbie (vitreous)
707 North Fairbanks Court
Chicago, Illinois 60611

Director of retina service, Northwestern University Medical School.

Dr. J. Donald Gass
Bascom-Palmer Eye Institute
University of Miami Medical School
1638 NW Tenth Avenue
Miami, Florida 33136

Professor of ophthalmology.

Dr. Froncie A. Gutman (vitreous)
Cleveland Clinic
Cleveland, Ohio 44106

Dr. William S. Hagler
2004 Peachtree Road, NE
Atlanta, Georgia 30309

Associate professor of ophthalmology, Emory University.

Dr. Alexander R. Irvine (vitreous)
400 Parnassus Avenue
San Francisco, California 94143

Associate professor of ophthalmology, University of California.

Dr. William H. Jarrett II
2004 Peachtree Road, NE
Atlanta, Georgia 30309

Associate professor of ophthalmology, Emory University.

Dr. Otto H. Jungschaffer
12840 Riverside Drive
North Hollywood, California 91607

Associate clinical professor of ophthalmology, University of Southern California.

Dr. William H. Knobloch
University of Minnesota Hospital
Minneapolis, Minnesota 55455

Professor of ophthalmology.

Dr. Allan E. Kreiger (vitreous)
Jules Stein Eye Institute
University of California at Los
Angeles Medical Center
Los Angeles, California 90024

Dr. Francis A. L'Esperance, Jr.
1 East 71st Street
New York, New York 10021

*Associate professor of clinical
ophthalmology, Columbia.*

Dr. Robert Machemer (vitreous)
Duke Medical Center
Durham, North Carolina 27710

*Professor of ophthalmology. Noted
for his refinement and
modernization of vitreous surgery.*

Dr. Edward B. McLean
Department of Ophthalmology
University of Washington Medical
School
Seattle, Washington 98195

Professor of ophthalmology.

Dr. Alice R. McPherson (vitreous)
Medical Center Professional
Building
6436 Fannin Street
Houston, Texas 77030

*Clinical associate professor of
ophthalmology, Baylor.*

Dr. David Meyer
1331 Union Avenue
Memphis, Tennessee 38104

*Clinical associate professor of
ophthalmology, University of
Tennessee.*

Dr. Lemuel T. Moorman (vitreous)
2045 Franklin Street
Denver, Colorado 80205

*Assistant clinical professor of
ophthalmology, University of
Colorado.*

Dr. Edward W. D. Norton
Bascom-Palmer Eye Institute
University of Miami Medical
School
1638 NW Tenth Avenue
Miami, Florida 33136

*Professor and chairman, department
of ophthalmology.*

Dr. Edward Okun
4989 Barnes Hospital Plaza
St. Louis, Missouri 63110

*Associate professor of
ophthalmology, Washington
University.*

Dr. Conor C. O'Malley (vitreous)
220 Meridian Road
San Jose, California 95126

*Associate clinical professor of
ophthalmology, University of
California.*

Dr. Stephen S. Pappas
6410 Rockledge Drive
Bethesda, Maryland 20034

*Clinical instructor in ophthalmology,
George Washington University.*

Dr. Arnall Patz
Wilmer Eye Institute
The Johns Hopkins Hospital
Baltimore, Maryland 21205

*Director of Retinal Vascular
Center. Professor and chairman,
department of ophthalmology.*

Dr. Charles D. J. Regan
Massachusetts Eye and Ear
Infirmary
243 Charles Street
Boston, Massachusetts 02114

*Associate professor of
ophthalmology, Harvard.*

Retina Associates
100 Charles River Plaza at
Cambridge Street
Boston, Massachusetts 02114

*Dr. Charles L. Schepens, director, is
a major figure in retina surgery.
All retina specialists at Retina
Associates are considered excellent.*

Dr. Dennis M. Robertson
Mayo Clinic
Rochester, Minnesota 55901

Dr. Richard Ruiz
Herman Eye Institute
University of Texas Medical
Center
Houston, Texas 77025

*Clinical associate professor of
ophthalmology, University of
Texas.*

Dr. Stephen J. Ryan
Doheny Eye Foundation
1355 San Pablo Street
Los Angeles, California 90033

*Professor and chairman, department
of ophthalmology, Southern
California University Medical
School.*

Dr. Felix N. Sabates
6700 Troost Avenue
Kansas City, Missouri 64131

*Chief of ophthalmology, University
of Missouri.*

Dr. Ariah Schwartz
1515 Trousdale Drive
Burlingame, California 94010

*Clinical professor of
ophthalmology, University of
California at Los Angeles.*

Dr. W. B. Snyder (vitreous)
5421 La Sierra
Dallas, Texas 75231

In private practice.

Dr. Bradley R. Straatsma
Jules Stein Eye Institute
University of California at Los
Angeles Medical Center
Los Angeles, California 90024

*Chairman, department of
ophthalmology; director of the
Jules Stein Eye Institute.*

Dr. William Tasman
Wills Eye Hospital
1601 Spring Garden Street
Philadelphia, Pennsylvania 19130

Dr. Robert C. Watzke
Department of Ophthalmology
University of Iowa Medical School
Iowa City, Iowa 52242

Professor of ophthalmology.

Dr. Robert B. Welch
Wilmer Eye Institute
The Johns Hopkins Hospital
Baltimore, Maryland 21205

*Co-director of the Retina Clinic at
the Wilmer Eye Institute.*

OPHTHALMIC PLASTIC SURGEONS

Dr. Henry I. Baylis
5400 Balboa Street
Encino, California 91316

Dr. George F. Buerger, Jr.
3520 Fifth Avenue
Suite 401
Pittsburgh, Pennsylvania 15213
Senior medical staff at Pittsburgh Eye and Ear Hospital.

Dr. Arthur Grove
Massachusetts Eye and Ear
Infirmary
243 Charles Street
Boston, Massachusetts 02114

Assistant professor of ophthalmology, Harvard. A special interest in tumors of the eyelids and diseases of the eye orbit.

Dr. Charles R. Leone, Jr.
504 Madison Square
San Antonio, Texas 78215

Associate professor of ophthalmology, University of Texas at San Antonio.

Dr. Clinton D. McCord
2004 Peachtree Street NE
Atlanta, Georgia 30309

Associate professor of ophthalmology, Emory University Medical School.

Dr. Charles M. Stephenson
850 Prospect Street
La Jolla, California 92037

Associate clinical professor of ophthalmology, University of California at San Diego.

Dr. Richard R. Tenzel
1100 NE 163rd Street
North Miami Beach, Florida 33162

Clinical professor of ophthalmology, University of Miami Medical School. A special interest in eyelid surgery and surgery of the tear duct system.

Dr. Stephen L. Trokel
Columbia-Presbyterian Medical
Center
635 West 165th Street
New York, New York 10032

Associate professor of ophthalmology.

Dr. Eugene Wiggs
1825 Gilpin Street
Denver, Colorado 80218

Clinical professor of ophthalmology, Colorado. Has a special interest in tumor surgery in the orbit, and in plastic surgery in the orbit.

Dr. Robert Wilkins
1121 Hermann Professional
Building
Houston, Texas 77025

Clinical associate professor of ophthalmology, University of Texas Medical School. Has a special interest in cosmetic surgery.

NEURO-OPHTHALMOLOGISTS

Dr. Melvin G. Alper
5454 Wisconsin Avenue
Chevy Chase, Maryland 20015

*Clinical professor of neuro-
ophthalmology, George
Washington Medical School.*

Dr. Richard Appen
1025 Regent Street
Madison, Wisconsin 53715

Dr. Mylesa M. Behrens
Columbia-Presbyterian Medical
Center
625 West 165th Street
New York, New York 10032

*Associate clinical professor of
ophthalmology.*

Dr. Ronald M. Burde
Washington University Medical
School
660 South Euclid
St. Louis, Missouri 63110

*Professor of ophthalmology and
neurology.*

Dr. David Cogan
Building 10
Room 13S261
National Institutes of Health
Bethesda, Maryland 20014

*Like all National Institutes of
Health patient care, there is no fee.
However, in order to be qualified
you require the referral of your
attending physician and you must
meet the National Institutes of
Health research protocols for your
particular disorder. Dr. Cogan does
consulting only.*

Dr. Robert B. Daroff
University of Miami Medical
School
Biscayne Annex
Miami, Florida 33152

Professor of ophthalmology.

Dr. Carl Ellenberger
Hershey Medical Center
Hershey, Pennsylvania 17033

Dr. Andrew J. Gay
Little River House
Belfast, Maine 04915

Dr. Joel S. Glaser
Bascom-Palmer Eye Institute
University of Miami Medical
School
Miami, Florida 33136

Dr. Thomas R. Hedges
Pennsylvania Hospital
Eighth and Spruce Streets
Philadelphia, Pennsylvania 19107

Professor of ophthalmology.

Dr. Robert S. Hepler
Jules Stein Eye Institute
University of California at Los
Angeles Medical Center
Los Angeles, California 90024

Professor of ophthalmology.

Dr. Robert Holtenhorst
Mayo Clinic
Rochester, Minnesota 55901

Professor of ophthalmology, Mayo.

Dr. William F. Hoyt
Neuro-Ophthalmology Unit
Moffitt Hospital
San Francisco, California 94143

*Professor of ophthalmology,
neurology, and neurosurgery,
University of California.*

Dr. Thomas Kearns
Mayo Clinic
Rochester, Minnesota 55901

Professor of ophthalmology, Mayo.

Dr. John L. Keltner
University of California at Davis
Davis, California 95616

*Chairman, department of
ophthalmology.*

Dr. John S. Kennerdal
Eye and Ear Hospital
230 Lothrop Street
Pittsburgh, Pennsylvania 15213

Dr. David Knox
The Johns Hopkins Hospital
Baltimore, Maryland 21205

*Associate professor of
ophthalmology.*

Dr. Simmons Lessell
750 Harrison Avenue
Boston, Massachusetts 02118

*Associate professor of neurology
and ophthalmology, Boston
University.*

Dr. Neil Miller
The Johns Hopkins Hospital
Baltimore, Maryland 21205

*Assistant professor of neurology
and ophthalmology.*

Dr. Nancy M. Newman
Pacific Medical Center
San Francisco, California 94115

*Assistant clinical professor of
ophthalmology, University of
California; head of neuro-
ophthalmology, Pacific Medical
Center.*

Dr. Joel G. Sacks
Medical Science Building
University of Cincinnati Medical
School
Cincinnati, Ohio 45267

*Chairman, department of
ophthalmology.*

Dr. J. Lawton Smith
Bascom-Palmer Eye Institute
University of Miami Medical
School
Miami, Florida 33136

Professor of ophthalmology.

Dr. H. Stanley Thompson
University of Iowa Hospitals
Iowa City, Iowa 52242

Professor of ophthalmology.

Dr. Jonathan D. Trobe
University of Florida Medical
School
Gainesville, Florida 32611

*Assistant professor of
ophthalmology.*

Dr. Henry J. L. Van Dyk
University of Utah Medical Center
Salt Lake City, Utah 84132

*Chairman, department of
ophthalmology, associate professor
of neurology.*

Dr. Thomas J. Walsh
1100 Bedford Street
Stamford, Connecticut 06905

*Associate clinical professor of
neurology and ophthalmology,
Yale.*

Dr. Shirley Wray
Massachusetts Eye and Ear
Infirmary
243 Charles Street
Boston, Massachusetts 02114

*Associate professor of
ophthalmology, Harvard.*

Dr. Robert D. Yee
Harbor General Hospital
Torrance, California 90509

Chief of ophthalmology.

Dr. David Zee
The Johns Hopkins Hospital
Baltimore, Maryland 21205

*Assistant professor of neurology
and ophthalmology.*

Diseases of the
Ear, Nose, and Throat

Subspecialties of Otolaryngology

Otolaryngologists are surgeons of the ear, nose, throat, and head and neck systems. Because of the separate functions of these regions of the body, otolaryngologists tend to subspecialize or have special interests in certain areas or certain surgical procedures. These are the general categories in which ear, nose, throat, and head and neck specialists have special or exclusive interests:

Head and neck cancer surgery. The vast preponderance of surgery in this region is for malignant tumors, although there are some operations that do not involve cancer. This surgery involves the area around the ear, the jaws, the neck, and the larnyx.

Ear tumors. Both otolaryngologists and neurosurgeons operate on ear tumors. Although the dividing line is not exact as to when one specialty performs the surgery and the other does not, in most cases when the tumor can be removed through the ear, the otolaryngologists perform it, and when the tumor requires removal through the head itself, neurosurgeons perform the surgery.

Middle ear. Infections, tumors, and other disorders can cause a rupture of the eardrum, hearing loss, and discharge, and necessitate surgery which in many cases will offer some restoration of hearing. Also, developmental defects and hereditary deafness problems can often be corrected through surgery.

Taste and smell. Although otolaryngology involves disorders of the nose and throat, there is little in the way of patient service for these relatively common disorders because so few physicians have specialized in them. It is estimated that perhaps five million Americans suffer some impairment of their taste or smell—either a metallic taste, or "burning tongue," or severe distortion of taste or smell or, in some cases, an absence of either—but few medical specialists have investigated these disorders. Such taste and smell disorders can result from the aftermath of an influenza virus, head injury, allergies, or radiation therapy to the region of the head and neck. One otolaryngologist has an interest in these disorders, and two centers, one chiefly a research center and the other a patient care center, deal with people with taste and smell disorders.

Vestibular disorders. Both dizziness and difficulties with balance can be caused by inner ear problems, and some specialists on this list have a special interest in these disorders.

Deafness. The cochlear implant, pioneered by Dr. William House, has allowed formerly deaf people to pick up "environmental noise." They cannot discriminate sounds well, but they can hear noise, such as horns beeping. They cannot distinguish words, however.

Facial paralysis. Facial pain and paralysis caused by a disorder to a nerve which reaches into the inner ear is a surgical specialty of some otolaryngologists.

Ménière's disease. A rare disease of the ear which causes vertigo, tinnitus, nausea, vomiting, and progressive deafness.

Stapes surgery. The bone stapes, located in the ear, can be affected by disease or injury and can cause hearing loss. There are surgical procedures which correct it.

Ear pain. Neurotology, a specialty concerned with the nerves in and around the ear, involves surgery to relieve ear pain caused by neurological disorders in this region.

Voice disorders and larynx reconstruction. Disorders of the voice are of special interest to some otolaryngologists. They are related to larynx reconstruction because the larynx contains the vocal cords.

Reconstructive ear surgery. The reconstruction of the ear and surrounding tissue after an accident, after tumor surgery, or because of a condition due to developmental (congenital) defects is a special interest of some otolaryngologists. It combines some of the techniques of plastic surgery and otolaryngology.

Hearing disorders. Although these can include a partial loss of hearing, they also include such problems as constant ringing in the ears (tinnitus) or a persistent high frequency sound.

Although most of the outstanding otolaryngologists listed here have some special interests, many of them have a more general medical practice in disorders of the ear, nose, and throat. Some, in fact, prefer to remain generalists.

OTOLARYNGOLOGISTS

Dr. Bobby R. Alford (tumors; hearing disorders; head and neck)
Department of Otolaryngology
Baylor Medical College
Houston, Texas 77025

Professor and chairman, department of otolaryngology. A special interest in neurological problems with the ear, and salivary glands.

Dr. David F. Austin (reconstructive ear surgery)
55 East Washington
Chicago, Illinois 60602

Associate professor of otolaryngology, University of Illinois Medical School.

Dr. Hugh Barber (vestibular disorders)
Toronto General Hospital
Toronto, Ontario
Canada M5G 1L7

Dr. Bloyce Hill Britton, Jr. (ear tumors; hearing disorders)
1300 North Vermont Street
Los Angeles, California 90027

Private practice.

Dr. James Ryan Chandler, Jr. (head and neck)
Department of Otolaryngology
Jackson Memorial Hospital
1776 NW Tenth Avenue
Miami, Florida 33152

Professor and chairman, department of otolaryngology, University of Miami Medical School.

Dr. G. Thane Cody (chronic ear disease)
Mayo Clinic
200 First Street, SW
Rochester, Minnesota 55901

Professor of otolaryngology, Mayo.

Dr. James A. Crabtree (middle ear)
1300 North Vermont
Los Angeles, California 90027

Clinical professor of medicine, University of Southern California.

Dr. Charles Cummings
University of Washington Medical School
Seattle, Washington 98195

Professor of otolaryngology.

Dr. J. Brown Farrior
(reconstructive ear surgery)
509 Bay Street
Tampa, Florida 33606

*Clinical professor of surgery and
chief of the section on
otolaryngology, University of
Southern Florida.*

Dr. Richard Gacek (middle ear)
State University of New York
Syracuse, New York 13210

*Professor and chairman of
otolaryngology.*

Dr. Michael E. Glasscock III
(tumors; inner ear)
1811 State Street
Nashville, Tennessee 37203

*Clinical assistant professor of
surgery, Vanderbilt Medical
School.*

Dr. Robert Henkin (taste and
smell)
Center for Molecular Nutrition and
Sensory Disorders
Georgetown University Hospital
Washington, District of Columbia
20007

*Dr. Henkin is an endocrinologist,
not an otolaryngologist, but is
listed here because this unit is the
only one in this country which treats
patients on a regular basis for smell
and taste disorders.*

Dr. William House (tumor)
Otological Medical Group
2122 West Third Street
Los Angeles, California 90057

*A well-known ear surgeon. Pioneer
of the cochlear implant, among
other innovations. Clinical
professor of otolaryngology,
University of Southern California
Medical School.*

Dr. William Hudson (general)
Duke Medical Center
Durham, North Carolina 27710

Professor of otolaryngology.

Dr. Richard Jesse (head and neck)
M. D. Anderson Hospital and
Tumor Institute
Houston, Texas 77030

*Dr. Jesse is not an otolaryngologist,
but is especially skilled in head
and neck tumor problems.*

Dr. Morley Kare, director
Monell Chemical Senses Center
3500 Market Street
Philadelphia, Pennsylvania 19104

*Affiliated with the University of
Pennsylvania Medical School. Dr.
Kare is not a medical doctor but is
director of this center, which is
long noted for its research into
taste and smell disorders. The
center does limited testing and
treatment of persons with taste and
smell disorders.*

Dr. Samuel Kinney (tumor and
middle ear)
Cleveland Clinic
Cleveland, Ohio 44106

Dr. Brian F. McCabe (middle ear)
University Hospital
Iowa City, Iowa 52242

Head of otolaryngology and maxillofacial surgery, University of Iowa Medical School.

Dr. Mark May (facial nerve)
3600 Frobest Avenue
Pittsburgh, Pennsylvania 15213

Dr. May also has an interest in taste and smell disorders.

Dr. William Montgomery (head and neck)
Massachusetts Eye and Ear Infirmary
243 Charles Street
Boston, Massachusetts 02114

Professor of otolaryngology, Harvard.

Dr. Eugene Myers (head and neck)
University of Pittsburgh Medical School
Pittsburgh, Pennsylvania 15213

Professor of otolaryngology.

Dr. George Nager (middle ear)
Johns Hopkins Hospital
Baltimore, Maryland 21205

Professor and chairman, department of laryngology and otolaryngology. Known also for his diagnostic interests.

Dr. Alvin J. Novack (head and neck)
1221 Madison Street
Seattle, Washington 98104

Clinical professor of otolaryngology, University of Washington.

Dr. Joseph Ogura (head and neck)
4959 Barnes Hospital Plaza
St. Louis, Missouri 63110

Lindberg professor and head, department of otolaryngology, Washington University.

Dr. Jack L. Pulec (ear diseases; pain control)
2161 Wilshire Boulevard
Los Angeles, California 90017

Associate clinical professor of otolaryngology, University of Southern California. Noted for his special interest in neurological problems of the ear.

Dr. William Saunders (general and middle ear)
University Hospital
Columbus, Ohio 43210

Chairman, department of otolaryngology, Ohio State.

Dr. Harold Schuknecht (Stapes surgery; middle ear)
Massachusetts Eye and Ear Infirmary
243 Charles Street
Boston, Massachusetts 02114

Professor of otolaryngology, Harvard.

Dr. John J. Shea, Jr.
(Stapes surgery)
Memphis Eye and Ear Hospital
1080 Madison Avenue
Memphis, Tennessee 38104

Founder of the Memphis Eye and Ear Hospital.

Dr. Herbert Silverstein (Ménière's disease)
1849 A Hawthorne
Sarasota, Florida 33579

Dr. George Sisson (head and neck)
Northwestern University Medical School
303 East Chicago Avenue
Chicago, Illinois 60611

Professor and chairman, department of otolaryngology and maxillofacial surgery.

Dr. Gershon Spector (head and neck)
Washington University Medical School
St. Louis, Missouri 63110

Professor of otolaryngology. Also known for ear surgery and middle ear surgery.

Dr. S. M. Strong (head and neck)
University Hospital
Boston, Massachusetts 02118

Professor of otolaryngology, Boston University; chief of otolaryngology service, University Hospital.

Dr. Howard Tabb (middle ear)
Tulane University Medical School
New Orleans, Louisiana 70112

Professor and chairman of otolaryngology.

Dr. Harvey Tucker
(larynx reconstruction)
Cleveland Clinic
Cleveland, Ohio 44106

Chairman, department of otolaryngology. Also noted for head and neck surgery.

Dr. Paul Ward (head and neck; vestibular and voice disorders)
University of California at Los Angeles Medical Center
Los Angeles, California 90024

Professor of surgery; chairman of head and neck surgery department.

Endocrinology

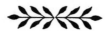

Endocrinologists

The endocrine system is composed of a complex system of hormone secreting glands in different parts of the body that are responsible for a number of vital human functions. The insulin producing cells of the pancreas are the most widely known parts of this system largely because a malfunction in these results in diabetes. Although diabetes specialists are also endocrinologists, there are some endocrinologists who specialize in the other parts of the endocrine system. It is within these endocrine glands that other vital human functions take place.

In brief, these are the major glands endocrine specialists are most involved with.

1. *The thyroid gland*. Located in the neck on either side of the trachea, this gland regulates the metabolism of the body. An overactive thyroid (hyperthyroidism) can cause severe weight loss, nervousness, agitation, eye disorders, and other problems. Hypothyroidism (an underactive thyroid) can cause weight gain, lethargy, growth disorders in children, and other problems.

2. *The parathyroid glands*. Located around the thyroid, these are a collection of very small glands (each about the size of a pea) which regulate the flow of calcium in the blood. A disorder of the para-

thyroid glands can cause bone diseases (from an excess or deficit of calcium) as well as kidney stones and other disorders.

3. *The pituitary gland.* Located in the base of the brain it is the master hormonal gland in the human body. It acts as the link between the nervous system and the rest of the endocrine glands. The pituitary gland plays a vital role in a number of important functions, but its major overall function is the regulation of the other endocrine glands. Disorders of the pituitary gland can result in a broad spectrum of symptoms and disorders.

4. *The reproductive glands.* Reproductive endocrinologists, a board certified subspecialty of obstetrics and gynecology, generally deal with women's reproductive problems. Endocrinologists, however, generally deal with men's reproductive glands and female gonadal dysfunction.

5. *The adrenal glands.* Located near the kidneys, the adrenal glands perform a number of functions. They produce adrenaline, which constricts the small blood vessels of the skin and elsewhere and raises the blood pressure and energy level when secreted quickly into the bloodstream. Cortisone is also produced by the adrenal glands, and when it is overproduced (by tumor or other disorder) it causes a disorder known as Cushing's disease which causes the face to become full and can also cause changes in the skin. High blood pressure can also result from adrenal tumors.

Another widely known disease associated with the endocrine glands is *Addison's disease.* Like Cushing's disease, it involves the adrenal glands. Low blood pressure, a brownish discoloration of the skin, and weakness are among the symptoms.

Sophisticated blood tests can usually determine with precision the type and extent of the hormonal problem, and because of these tests, one endocrinologist remarked, "we know a lot more about the endocrine system than we know about other parts of the body."

It should be noted here that those lymph glands you feel in your neck, especially when they swell due to an infection, are not part of the endocrine system. The endocrine glands include only those glands which secrete hormones. The lymph glands essentially serve to collect and dispose of germs and other debris in the body.

Endocrinologists treat all endocrine problems, but like other specialists, some endocrinologists are known for their special interests and their special areas of research. Those with established special interests are so noted. Endocrinologists noted for their diabetes work are listed in the diabetes section. However, in some cases some specialists do clinical care in both diabetes and general endocrinology.

ENDOCRINOLOGISTS

Dr. Louis Avioli (bone diseases)
Jewish Hospital of St. Louis
St. Louis, Missouri 63110

Professor of medicine, Washington University Medical School.

Dr. David Becker (thyroid)
New York Hospital–Cornell
Medical Center
525 East 68th Street
New York, New York 10021

Professor of medicine and radiology; director, division of nuclear medicine. As noted in the nuclear medicine section, some nuclear medicine specialists subspecialize in thyroid disorders, including thyroid cancer.

Dr. William H. Beierwaltes
(thyroid)
Department of Nuclear Medicine
University of Michigan
Medical Center
Ann Arbor, Michigan 48104

Professor of internal medicine; director of nuclear medicine division.

Dr. A. Richard Christlieb
(adrenal hypertension problems)
Joslin Clinic
1 Joslin Place
Boston, Massachusetts 02215

Dr. Nicholas P. Christy (adrenal)
Roosevelt Hospital
428 West 59th Street
New York, New York 10019

Professor of medicine, Columbia.

Dr. Eugene P. Clerkin
Lahey Clinic
605 Commonwealth Avenue
Boston, Massachusetts 02215

Dr. William Daughaday (pituitary)
Barnes Hospital Plaza
St. Louis, Missouri 63110

*Professor of medicine,
Washington University.*

Dr. Leslie J. DeGroot (thyroid)
University of Chicago Hospitals
950 East 59th Street
Chicago, Illinois 60637

Professor of medicine.

Dr. Philip R. Eaton
University of New Mexico
Medical School
Albuquerque, New Mexico 87131

Professor of medicine.

Dr. Stefan Fajans
Endocrinology and
Metabolism Clinic
University of Michigan
Medical Center
Ann Arbor, Michigan 48109

Professor of medicine.

Dr. Daniel D. Federman
Massachusetts General Hospital
Boston, Massachusetts 02214

Professor of medicine, Harvard.

Dr. James Fields
Baylor College of Medicine
Houston, Texas 77025

Professor of medicine.

Dr. Norbert Freinkel
Center for Endocrinology,
Metabolism and Nutrition
Northwestern University
Medical School
303 East Chicago Avenue
Chicago, Illinois 60611

Director of center.

Dr. Clifford F. Gastineau
Mayo Clinic
Rochester, Minnesota 55901

Professor of medicine, Mayo.

Dr. Francis S. Greenspan (thyroid)
University of California
Medical School
San Francisco, California 94143

*Clinical professor of medicine, chief
of thyroid clinic.*

Dr. John Hare (thyroid)
Joslin Clinic
1 Joslin Place
Boston, Massachusetts 02215

Dr. Dorothy T. Krieger
Mt. Sinai Medical School
1 East 100th Street
New York, New York 10028

Professor of medicine.

Dr. Joseph Kriss (thyroid)
Stanford University Medical Center
Stanford, California 94305

*Director of nuclear medicine.
Known for his special interest
in thyroid.*

Dr. Grant Liddle
(Cushing's disease)
Vanderbilt Medical Center
Nashville, Tennessee 37232

Professor of medicine.

Dr. James C. Melby
Boston University Medical Center
80 East Concord Street
Boston, Massachusetts 02118

Professor of medicine.

Dr. Thomas Merimee
University of Florida
Medical School
Gainesville, Florida 32601

*Chief, division of endocrinology
and metabolism.*

Dr. Robert L. Ney
Department of Medicine
University of North Carolina
Medical School
Chapel Hill, North Carolina 27514

*Professor and chairman, department
of medicine.*

Dr. Charles A. Nugent (adrenal)
University of Arizona
Medical School
Tucson, Arizona 85724

Professor of internal medicine.

Dr. William D. O'Dell
Harbor General Hospital
Torrance, California 90509

*Professor and chairman, department
of medicine, University of California
at Los Angeles.*

Dr. Jack Oppenheimer (thyroid)
University of Miami Medical School
Biscayne Annex
Miami, Florida 33152

Professor of medicine.

Dr. David N. Orth
Vanderbilt Medical Center
Nashville, Tennessee 37232

Professor of medicine.

Dr. Seymour Reichlin
(neuroendocrinology)
New England Medical Center
171 Harrison Avenue
Boston, Massachusetts 02111

*Professor of medicine, Tufts.
Neuroendocrinology deals with the
relationship between the nervous
system and the endocrine system.
Many problems in this area
involve the pituitary gland and
can result in a number of different
disorders and symptoms. Dr.
Reichlin is a recognized leader in
this area.*

Dr. Eric Reiss (parathyroid)
University of Miami Medical School
Biscayne Annex
Miami, Florida 33152

*Professor and chairman, department
of medicine.*

Dr. Robert Salasa (pituitary)
Mayo Clinic
Rochester, Minnesota 55901

Professor of medicine, Mayo.

Dr. Naguib Samaan (pituitary)
M. D. Anderson Hospital and
Tumor Institute
6723 Bertner Avenue
Houston, Texas 77030

*Chief, section on endocrinology;
professor of internal medicine,
Baylor.*

Dr. Theodore B. Schwartz
Rush Presbyterian–St. Luke's
Medical Center
1753 West Congress Parkway
Chicago, Illinois 60660

*Professor and chairman, department
of medicine, Rush Medical College.*

Dr. Penn Skillern
Cleveland Clinic
Cleveland, Ohio 44106

Chief of endocrinology.

Dr. Peter Snyder (thyroid)
University of Pennsylvania
Medical School
522 Johnson Pavilion
Philadelphia, Pennsylvania 19104

Assistant professor of medicine.

Dr. David H. Solomon
University of California at Los
Angeles Medical Center
Los Angeles, California 90024

Chairman, department of medicine.

Adult Diabetes

The listings of diabetes specialists are divided between adult and
juvenile specialists.* However, many of those specialists appearing on

* Specialists in juvenile diabetes are listed in Part III, under the section "Endocrine
Disorders."

the juvenile diabetes list also handle adult cases. The opposite is generally not true. Adult diabetes specialists as a rule do not handle juvenile diabetes cases. Thus, if you are an adult diabetic the listings for both juvenile and adult specialists can be useful. If you need assistance in juvenile diabetes, consult the juvenile list *only*. It should be noted that those juvenile diabetes specialists who are pediatricians or who are attached to children's hospitals do *not* see adult patients.

One reason for this division is that medical management of juvenile and adult diabetes is very different. Some physicians, in fact, regard adult and juvenile diabetes as two different diseases. Juvenile diabetes is generally a more virulent disease. It almost always requires insulin injections and other radical treatments, while adult onset diabetes can often be treated effectively by weight loss and diet alone. However, many adults obviously have juvenile-*type* diabetes, having been diagnosed with the disease when they were young.

Diabetes, especially juvenile-type, is a very difficult disease to treat and manage properly. In the words of a leading diabetes specialist, "It is very easy for diabetes management to be bad. To be an expert," he continued, "you should be treating it day in and day out. It requires considerable experience. There is quite a lot of art to good diabetes management."

He cited several ways in which diabetes can be poorly managed.

1. Some people are on oral hypoglycemic drugs rather than insulin injections.
2. Some physicians do not know how to adjust the insulin level properly.
3. Many overweight diabetics are treated needlessly with insulin. Diet therapy alone is often preferable.
4. The patient and the patient's family must be trained to live with diabetes. This is sometimes neglected.
5. Some physicians do not readily admit when a diabetic case, especially one in which the management is very tricky, is beyond them. Thus, the patient suffers needlessly.

As diabetes becomes more prevalent—some 5 percent of the U.S. population has it—knowledge of the disease and its proper management is improving. But specialists report seeing many cases of poor management every year. One area of mismanagement and disagreement is the use of oral hypoglycemic drugs—drugs to reduce the high blood sugar associated with diabetes. Some specialists do not think these drugs have *any* place in diabetes treatment; others think they do have a place but are sometimes given to the wrong people. Also, the controversy over the role of the oral hypoglycemics in increasing the heart attack risk remains unsettled.

There is little question that a clinical trial showed diabetics who received one oral hypoglycemic drug did have a higher incidence of heart attack than those on insulin and placebo. However, some diabetologists argue that the study was not conclusive. The controversy remains. If oral hypoglycemics are used, a leading diabetes expert said, they should be used only for adult diabetics who do not have symptoms other than an elevated blood sugar. "I think there is a place for the oral drug," he said, "but it is a limited one." Others, of course, disagree.

ADULT DIABETES AND HYPOGLYCEMIA SPECIALISTS

Dr. John Bagdade
University of Washington
Seattle, Washington 98195

Associate professor of medicine.

Dr. Buris R. Boshell
Diabetes Hospital
1808 Seventh Avenue South
Birmingham, Alabama 35294

Professor of medicine; director of endocrinology and metabolic division, University of Alabama.

Dr. Robert Bradley
Joslin Clinic
1 Joslin Place
Boston, Massachusetts 02215

Dr. John J. Canary
Georgetown University
Medical School
3800 Reservoir Road, NW
Washington, District of Columbia
20007

Professor of medicine; chief of endocrinology and metabolic division.

Dr. Dana Clarke
Division of Metabolism
Clinical Research Center
University of Utah Medical Center
50 North Medical Drive
Salt Lake City, Utah 84132

Assistant professor of medicine; medical director of diabetes clinic.

Dr. John A. Colwell
171 Ashley Avenue
Charleston, South Carolina 29403

Professor of medicine, University of South Carolina; director of endocrinology and metabolic division.

Dr. John K. Davidson III
Emory University Hospital
Atlanta, Georgia 30322

Professor of medicine, chief of the diabetes unit.

Dr. Vincent DiRaimondo
4141 Geary Boulevard
Suite 201
San Francisco, California 94118

Dr. Harold L. Dobson
Hermann Hospital
Houston, Texas 77030

*Clinical associate professor of
medicine, Baylor; head of the
Diabetic Clinic, Hermann Hospital.*

Dr. Henry Dolger
11 East 86th Street
New York, New York 10028

*Director of the Diabetes Clinic,
Mt. Sinai.*

Dr. Max Ellenberg
936 Fifth Avenue
New York, New York 10021

*Clinical professor of medicine,
Mt. Sinai Medical School.*

Dr. Jerome M. Feldman
Duke Medical Center
Durham, North Carolina 27710

Professor of medicine.

Dr. Edmund B. Flink
Endocrinology Section
Medical Center of
West Virginia University
Morgantown, West Virginia 26506

*Professor and chairman, department
of medicine.*

Dr. Clifford F. Gastineau
The Mayo Clinic
Diabetes Unit
200 First Street, SW
Rochester, Minnesota 55901

Professor of medicine.

Dr. Saul Genuth
Mt. Sinai Hospital of Cleveland
Cleveland, Ohio 44106

*Associate professor of medicine,
Case-Western Reserve.*

Dr. Frederick C. Goetz
University of Minnesota Hospital
Minneapolis, Minnesota 55455

Dr. Harvey Hamff
478 Peachtree, NE
Atlanta, Georgia 30308

*Clinical professor of
medicine, Emory.*

Dr. John Karam
University of California
Medical Center
Third and Parnassus
San Francisco, California 94143

Associate professor of medicine.

Dr. Samuel D. Loube
2400 H Street, NW
Washington, District of Columbia
20037

*Clinical professor of medicine,
George Washington University.*

Dr. Richard J. Mahler
39000 Bob Hope Drive
Palm Desert, California 92260

*Director, department of metabolism
and endocrinology, Eisenhower
Medical Center.*

Dr. Daniel Mintz
University of Miami Medical School
Biscayne Annex
Miami, Florida 33152

Professor of medicine.

Dr. Robert Nielsen
Mason Clinic
Diabetes Unit
1100 Ninth Avenue
Seattle, Washington 98111

*Seattle is very strong in diabetes
care. Mason Clinic has a number
of superb diabetes specialists.*

Dr. Thaddeus Prout
Greater Baltimore Medical Center
6701 North Charles Street
Baltimore, Maryland 21204

Associate professor of medicine,
Johns Hopkins.

Dr. Harold Rifkin
35 East 75th Street
New York, New York 10021

Professor of clinical medicine,
New York University.

Dr. John W. Runyan
266 North Pauline
Memphis, Tennessee 38105

Professor and chairman, department
of community medicine, University
of Tennessee.

Dr. Penn G. Skillern
Cleveland Clinic
Cleveland, Ohio 44106

Chief of endocrinology.

Dr. T. Franklin Williams
Monroe Community Hospital
Rochester, New York 14603

Professor of medicine, preventive
medicine, and radiation biology,
University of Rochester.

Endocrine Surgeons

One of the newer surgical subspecialties is surgery of the endocrine glands. Specifically, endocrine surgeons specialize in surgery on the thyroid, adrenal glands, and parathyroid glands. Some concentrate on endocrine secreting pancreatic and bowel tumors as well, but this overlaps with gastrointestinal (GI) surgeons who concentrate on this same area. Some pancreatic endocrine tumors, for example, secrete hormones that result in severe hypoglycemia (low blood sugar concentrations), severe peptic ulcers, and even massive diarrhea. Removal of these tumors can completely cure these conditions in many instances.

Surgery on the pituitary gland is performed by neurosurgeons, and surgery on the reproductive glands is usually performed by urologists for men and reproductive endocrinologists, a subspecialty of obstetrics and gynecology, for women.

As in other areas of medicine, some endocrine surgeons concentrate on specific glands, and those with such special interests are so noted. Most endocrine surgeons are general surgeons who have specialized in endocrine surgery but also continue to perform general GI surgery.

The single most common type of endocrine surgery is performed on the thyroid gland. This surgery is performed for two main reasons: correction of an overactive hyperfunctioning thyroid gland (Graves' disease) or the evaluation and treatment of a lump in the thyroid since this might be a cancer.

There are techniques for surgical removal of part or all of the thyroid gland (its function can be assumed by hormones taken in pill form). For cases of hyperthyroidism, a removal of part of the thyroid gland is preferable, especially in young adults because of the uncertainties of using radioactive iodine treatment during the reproductive years.

Another major cause of the increase in thyroid surgery is thyroid cancer. There appears to be a significant increase in this disease in recent years. This increased prevalence is thought to be due to the fact that in the past many persons were given radiation therapy as treatment for tonsillitis, to shrink the thymus gland (thought to be the cause of sudden crib-deaths in infants), or to treat acne. These treatments are no longer done at major medical centers. The result of exposure of the thyroid gland to low-dose radiation appears to be clearly linked to a significant increase in thyroid cancer in these individuals. Studies in the past show that out of a population of one million, only thirty-six (.0036 percent) would be expected to have cancer of the thyroid. However, in the group of individuals who have had these low-dose radiation treatments to the neck area, up to 9 percent have been found to have cancer of the thyroid. This means that people radiated in the neck area in this manner have a much greater chance of getting thyroid cancer.

There are tumors in other areas of the endocrine system as well. Tumors of the adrenal glands can cause high blood pressure and an excess production of aldosterone, adrenaline, or cortisone. These tumors are especially important to diagnose because their presence can be life-threatening. Furthermore, the hypertension is usually reversible after their removal.

Tumors of the parathyroid glands cause an elevation of the calcium concentration in the blood. This can result in serious medical problems—kidney stones, bone thinning, peptic ulcers, arthritis, constipation, and many minor aches and pains. Removal of the enlarged gland or glands can result in a complete reversal of these events.

Endocrine surgery, according to one endocrine surgeon, "is often delicate and precise." He noted, for example, that many surgeons not experienced in parathyroid surgery might actually miss finding enlarged parathyroid glands or take out normal parathyroid glands without noticing them during thyroid surgery because the parathyroid glands are so small when normal and because changes associated with overactivity may be subtle. "Also," an endocrine surgeon noted, "there are very exacting decisions. When one operates to remove part of a thyroid that is overactive, how much tissue should be taken out and how much gland should be preserved? This is very important to that patient since his or her thyroid function might ultimately depend upon this. Furthermore, in thyroid surgery there is the risk of paralysis of the vocal cords if a small nerve passing near the thyroid gland is injured, a risk that is greatly minimized in the hands of an experienced neck surgeon. In general, the results of surgical procedures for hyperthyroidism and hyperparathyroidism are very good in the hands of experienced endocrine surgeons."

Following is a list of some of the most experienced and respected surgeons in the country in the field of endocrine surgery, which has far fewer specialists than many of the other specialties.

ENDOCRINE SURGEONS

Dr. Blake Cady
Lahey Clinic
605 Commonwealth Avenue
Boston, Massachusetts 02215

Assistant clinical professor of surgery, Harvard.

Dr. Orlo Clark
(thyroid, parathyroid)
University of California
Medical Center
San Francisco, California 94143

Assistant professor of surgery.

Dr. Anthony Edis (parathyroid)
Mayo Clinic
Rochester, Minnesota 55901

Dr. Richard H. Egdahl (adrenal)
Boston University Medical School
Boston, Massachusetts 02118

Professor, department of surgery.

Dr. Caldwell B. Esselstyn, Jr.
(thyroid, parathyroid)
Cleveland Clinic
Cleveland, Ohio 44106

Dr. Timothy S. Harrison
(adrenal tumors, insulin secreting
tumors of the pancreas)
Hershey Medical Center
Hershey, Pennsylvania 17033

Professor of surgery and physiology.

Dr. Edwin Kaplan (thyroid,
parathyroid endocrine tumors
of the GI tract)
University of Chicago Hospitals
950 East 59th Street
Chicago, Illinois 60637

*Professor of surgery, University
of Chicago Medical School.*

Dr. Edward Paloyan
(parathyroid, thyroid)
Loyola University School of
Medicine
2160 South First Avenue
Maywood, Illinois 60153

Professor of surgery.

Dr. Colin G. Thomas, Jr.
(thyroid)
University of North Carolina
Medical School
Chapel Hill, North Carolina 27514

Professor of surgery.

Dr. Norman W. Thompson
(thyroid, parathyroid)
University of Michigan
Medical Center
Ann Arbor, Michigan 48104

Professor of surgery.

Dr. Chiu-An Wang
(parathyroid and thyroid)
Massachusetts General Hospital
Boston, Massachusetts 02114

*Associate clinical professor of
surgery, Harvard.*

Dr. Samuel A. Wells (parathyroid)
Duke Medical Center
Durham, North Carolina 27710

*Associate professor of surgery.
Dr. Wells is a pioneer in the
transplantation of parathyroid
tissue from the neck to the
arm muscle, a successful
procedure now widely adopted
for patients with secondary
hyperparathyroidism.*

Digestive Disease Specialists

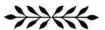

Gastroenterologists

Digestive diseases affect eighteen million Americans and are the cause
of more people going to the hospital than any other group of disorders.
Thirty percent of all cancers involve the digestive organs, and a number of other disorders, including ulcers, colitis, and gallstones, cause
many people serious and often debilitating illness.

A major problem in digestive disorders is to separate "functional
problems" from real organic disease. Functional problems—problems
which can cause discomfort but are not caused by any organic disease
—often result in extensive diagnostic tests being taken before they are
identified.

A number of new technologies now exist which greatly aid gastroenterologists in determining whether there is organic digestive disease.
Liver scans, arteriography, and endoscopy are often used. In fact,
says one prominent gastroenterologist, "the endoscope is terribly overused. I think," he continued, "there are a lot of pressures which cause
it to be overused. First, the patients have heard about it and they want
it used on them so they can have the benefit of the most modern diagnostic tool; second, the doctors who refer to specialists expect us to use
it; and finally, insurance pays for it."

The fiberoptic endoscope, which is certainly one of the major breakthroughs in diagnostic medicine in the past several years, is a small, flexible tube which can be fed into the digestive system and passed all through it to allow close-up visualization of any abnormal changes. While very useful, many endoscopic examinations are done with minimal indications. The better gastroenterologists, of course, only use the endoscope when there are clear and convincing indications for it.

Gastroenterologists deal with the full range of digestive problems. However, some gastroenterologists have subspecialized in liver disorders, and because they do this exclusively they appear on a separate list. Those gastroenterologists not specializing in liver diseases generally specialize in digestive diseases. They diagnose and medically treat problems of the digestive system. The major diseases diagnosed and treated in gastroenterology are:

1. *GI cancer.* Diagnosis and treatment, especially of the colon, stomach, and pancreas.

2. *Pancreatic problems.* Such as acute and chronic pancreatitis, and pancreatic cancer, which is increasing in incidence.

3. *Inflammatory bowel disease.* Also called Crohn's disease and ulcerative colitis. Inflammatory bowel disease may involve the large bowel or small bowel.

4. *Ulcers.* Diagnosis and treatment. There are a number of alternative treatments to peptic ulcers. Drug treatment, including drugs which depress acid formation, as well as a surgical technique called vagotomy, have all improved medical approaches to ulcers.

5. *Esophagea problems.* Hiatal hernias, peptic esophagitis, and dysphagia (having trouble swallowing) are some of the esophageal problems gastroenterologists treat.

6. *Absorption problems.* The absorption of food and vital nutrients into the bloodstream occurs in the small bowel. Chronic bowel diseases such as diarrhea (the world's leading killer of infants and children) prevent the absorption of these nutrients into the body and cause malnutrition.

7. *Gallbladder and biliary passage diseases.* Several million Americans have gallstones. Besides surgical removal, there are promising ways to remove them without surgery.

The outstanding individuals listed here all practice the full range of gastroenterology. Some of them are chiefly consultants while others are more directly involved in day-to-day patient care.

GASTROENTEROLOGISTS

Dr. David H. Alpers
Washington University
Medical School
St. Louis, Missouri 63110

Professor of medicine.

Dr. Martin Brotman
655 Sutter Street
San Francisco, California 94102

*Associate clinical professor of
medicine, University of California.*

Dr. John Carbone
University of California
Medical Center
San Francisco, California 94143

Professor of medicine.

Dr. Robert M. Donaldson, Jr.
Yale University Medical School
New Haven, Connecticut 06510

Professor of medicine.

Dr. Richard G. Farmer
Cleveland Clinic
Cleveland, Ohio 44106

Chairman, department of medicine.

Dr. John T. Farrar
Medical College of Virginia
Richmond, Virginia 23298

Professor of medicine.

Dr. John S. Fordtran
Southwestern Medical School
Dallas, Texas 75235

*Professor of medicine; head of
gastroenterology at Southwestern
and Parkland Memorial Hospital.*

Dr. Norton J. Greenberger
University of Kansas
Medical Center
Kansas City, Kansas 66103

*Professor and chairman, department
of medicine.*

Dr. Thomas R. Hendrix
The Johns Hopkins Hospital
Baltimore, Maryland 21205

Associate professor of medicine.

Dr. Jon I. Isenberg
University of California at Los
Angeles Medical Center
Los Angeles, California 90024

*Chief of gastroenterology at the
Veterans Administration hospital;
associate professor of medicine at
University of California at
Los Angeles.*

Dr. Kurt J. Isselbacher
Massachusetts General Hospital
Boston, Massachusetts 02114

Professor of medicine at Harvard.

Dr. Henry D. Janowitz
1075 Park Avenue
New York, New York 10028

*Clinical professor of medicine
and head of gastroenterology,
Mt. Sinai Hospital.*

Dr. Fred Kern, Jr.
University of Colorado
Medical Center
Denver, Colorado 80262

*Head of gastroenterology; professor
of medicine. Also noted for his
interest in liver disorders.*

Dr. Joseph Kirsner
University of Chicago Hospitals
950 East 59th Street
Chicago, Illinois 60637

Professor of medicine.

Dr. Burton Korelitz
Lenox Hill Hospital
100 East 77th Street
New York, New York 10021

Chief of gastroenterology.

Dr. Clarence Ledgerton
Medical University Hospital
171 Ashley Avenue
Charleston, South Carolina 29403

*Professor of medicine and chief of
gastroenterology, University of
South Carolina.*

Dr. James E. McGuigan
University of Florida
Medical School
Gainesville, Florida 32601

*Professor of medicine; chief of
gastroenterology.*

Dr. Charles Moertel
Mayo Clinic
Rochester, Minnesota 55901

*Considered an authority on
GI cancer.*

Dr. F. Warren Nugent
Lahey Clinic
605 Commonwealth Avenue
Boston, Massachusetts 02215

Dr. Robert Peters
4864 North Van Ness
Fresno, California 93704

*Clinical professor of medicine,
University of California at
Los Angeles.*

Dr. Sidney Phillips
Mayo Clinic
Rochester, Minnesota 55901

*Professor of medicine,
Mayo Medical School.*

Dr. Irwin Rosenberg
University of Chicago Hospitals
950 East 59th Street
Chicago, Illinois 60637

*Head of gastroenterology;
professor of medicine.*

Dr. Cyrus Rubin
University of Washington
Medical School
Seattle, Washington 98195

Professor of medicine.

Dr. John T. Sessions, Jr.
University of North Carolina
Medical School
Chapel Hill, North Carolina 27514

Professor of medicine.

Dr. Howard Shapiro
University of California
Medical Center
Third and Parnassus
San Francisco, California 94143

Clinical professor of medicine.

Dr. Paul Sherlock
Memorial Hospital for Cancer and
Allied Diseases
1275 York Avenue
New York, New York 10021

*Professor of medicine, Cornell;
head of gastroenterology at
Memorial. An authority on
gastrointestinal cancer.*

Dr. Marvin H. Sleisenger
University of California
Medical Center
San Francisco, California 94143

Professor of medicine.

Dr. Konrad H. Soergel
Milwaukee County General Hospital
Milwaukee, Wisconsin 52226

*Chief of gastroenterology; and
professor of medicine, Wisconsin
Medical College.*

Dr. Howard Spiro
Yale University Medical School
New Haven, Connecticut 06510

Professor of medicine.

Dr. Johnson L. Thistle
Mayo Clinic
Rochester, Minnesota 55901

Dr. Jerry S. Trier
Peter Bent Brigham Hospital
Boston, Massachusetts 02115

*Associate professor of medicine,
Harvard; director, division of
gastroenterology, Peter Bent
Brigham.*

Dr. Malcolm Tyor
Duke Medical Center
Durham, North Carolina 27710

*Professor of medicine; chief of
gastroenterology.*

Dr. Richard Wechsler
220 Meyran Avenue
Pittsburgh, Pennsylvania 15213

*Clinical associate professor of
medicine, University of Pittsburgh.*

Dr. Elliot Weser
University of Texas Medical School
San Antonio, Texas 78284

Professor of medicine.

Dr. Charles S. Winans
University of Chicago Hospitals
950 East 59th Street
Chicago, Illinois 60637

Professor of medicine.

Dr. Sidney J. Winawer
Cornell University
College of Medicine
1275 York Avenue
New York, New York 10021

*Clinical associate professor of
medicine. An authority on
gastrointestinal cancer.*

Liver Specialists

Perhaps the two diseases most responsible for creating the demand
for liver specialists are hepatitis and alcoholism. Says one liver specialist: "The liver is a very complex organ. Although liver disease is
not a board certified subspecialty, it is a subspecialty in fact because
of its complexity."

Most of the liver specialists listed here do considerable research in
the causes and possible cures of liver disease, but they also consult on

complex liver cases. In addition, some also have ongoing interests in other digestive disorders.

LIVER SPECIALISTS

Dr. James Boyer
Yale University Medical School
New Haven, Connecticut 06510

Professor of medicine; head of the liver unit.

Dr. Burton Combes
Southwestern Medical School
5323 Harry Hines Boulevard
Dallas, Texas 75235

Professor of internal medicine.

Dr. Harold Fallon
Medical College of Virginia
Richmond, Virginia 23298

Professor and chairman, department of medicine.

Dr. John T. Galambos
Emory University Medical School
69 Butler Street
Atlanta, Georgia 30303

Professor of medicine. Not limited to liver diseases.

Dr. Roger Lester
University of Pittsburgh
Medical School
Pittsburgh, Pennsylvania 15213

Professor of medicine.

Dr. Douglas B. McGill
Mayo Clinic
Rochester, Minnesota 55901

Professor of medicine; chairman, division of gastroenterology. Not limited to liver diseases.

Dr. Willis C. Maddrey
The Johns Hopkins Hospital
Baltimore, Maryland 21205

Associate professor of medicine.

Dr. Allan Redeker
Los Angeles County–University of
Southern California Medical Center
Los Angeles, California 90033

Professor of medicine, University of Southern California. A special interest in hepatitis.

Dr. Telfer Reynolds
Los Angeles County–University of
Southern California Medical Center
1200 Broad Street
Los Angeles, California 90033

Professor of medicine, University of Southern California.

Dr. Fenton Schaffner
Mt. Sinai Hospital
100th Street and Fifth Avenue
New York, New York 10029

Professor of medicine, Mt. Sinai Medical School.

Dr. Steven Schenker
Vanderbilt Medical Center
Nashville, Tennessee 37203

Professor of medicine. Not limited to liver diseases.

Dr. Rudi Schmid
University of California
Medical Center
San Francisco, California 94143

Professor of medicine.

Gastrointestinal Surgeons

Gastrointestinal surgery is involved with the organs of the digestive system. All gastrointestinal surgeons are general surgeons who operate on all parts of the digestive system. There are no officially recognized subspecialties. However, as in other specialties, some gastrointestinal surgeons are noted for particular areas of expertise. These areas include:

Cancer. All gastrointestinal surgeons perform cancer surgery, which in fact makes up the bulk of their work. However, a few concentrate almost entirely in this area.

Colon and rectal surgery. Most gastrointestinal surgeons perform colon and rectal surgery, but some are more identified with it. Some are listed here because they also do other types of GI surgery. Others who specialize exclusively in colon and rectal surgery are listed in the colon and rectal surgery section.

Operations for obesity (gastric and intestinal by-pass). These procedures have the potential of being overused and abused for weight reduction. The intestinal by-pass in particular has been abused in this regard. Nevertheless, when skillfully done for correct indications, it serves a useful purpose for some people. As of now, the gastric by-pass rather than the intestinal by-pass enjoys more favor as an accepted surgical procedure.

Pancreas. Some GI surgeons are identified with pancreatic surgery and in fact many regard it as a subspecialty of GI surgery. Statistics in recent years indicate that pancreatic cancer is increasing substantially.

Liver and biliary tract. This is another area in which some GI surgeons have a special interest and which is an area some GI surgeons regard as a distinct subspecialty. For liver transplantation, see Kidney and Liver Transplantation.

Esophagus. Both GI and thoracic surgeons operate on the esophagus, and some physicians in both specialties are particularly known for their work in this area.

Stomach and duodenum. Again, some GI surgeons have a special interest in this area, and surgery in this region is often performed for cancer or ulcers.

Liver transplant. One physician also listed under Kidney and Liver Transplantation is named here for liver transplantation.

It should be emphasized that all of the surgeons listed here are general (gastrointestinal) surgeons and some of them are noted for their special surgical interests.

GASTROINTESTINAL SURGEONS

Dr. George Block (inflammatory bowel disease; colon cancer)
University of Chicago Hospitals
950 East 59th Street
Chicago, Illinois 60637

Professor of surgery.

Dr. Henry Buchwald (surgery for obesity and hyperlipemia)
University of Minnesota Hospital
Minneapolis, Minnesota 55455

Associate professor of medicine, Minnesota. Hyperlipemia means excessive cholesterol and triglyceride levels.

Dr. John Cameron (liver; biliary tract; pancreas)
The Johns Hopkins Hospital
Baltimore, Maryland 21205

Associate professor of surgery.

Dr. Larry Carey
University Hospital
410 West Tenth Avenue
Columbus, Ohio 43210

Professor and chairman, department of surgery.

Dr. Robert Condon (stomach; duodenum; pancreas; biliary tract)
Medical College of Wisconsin
Milwaukee, Wisconsin 53226

Professor of surgery.

Dr. Avram Cooperman (pancreas; liver)
Cleveland Clinic
Cleveland, Ohio 44106

Dr. Gerald DeCosse (GI cancer)
Hospital for Cancer and Allied Diseases
1275 York Avenue
New York, New York 10021

Dr. Lawrence Den Besten
University of California at Los Angeles Medical Center
Los Angeles, California 90024

Professor of surgery.

Dr. Josef Fischer
Department of Surgery
University of Cincinnati
Medical Center
Cincinnati, Ohio 45267

Professor of surgery.

Dr. Ward O. Griffen, Jr.
University of Kentucky
Medical Center
Lexington, Kentucky 40506

Professor and chairman of surgery.

Dr. George Hallenbeck
Scripps Clinic
La Jolla, California 92037

Chairman, department of surgery.

Dr. Robert Hermann
(pancreas; liver)
Cleveland Clinic
Cleveland, Ohio 44106

Dr. Rayford Scott Jones
Duke Medical Center
Durham, North Carolina 27707

Associate professor of surgery.

Dr. Paul Jordan
(esophagus; stomach)
Baylor College of Medicine
Houston, Texas 77030

Professor of surgery.

Dr. Keith Kelly (stomach)
Mayo Clinic
Rochester, Minnesota 55901

Dr. Walter Lawrence (GI cancer)
Medical College of Virginia
Richmond, Virginia 23298

*Professor and chairman, department
of surgery.*

Dr. William P. Longmire
(pancreas; liver; biliary tract)
University of California at Los
Angeles Medical Center
Los Angeles, California 90024

Professor of surgery.

Dr. Robert McClelland
University of Texas-Southwestern
Medical School
5323 Harry Hines Boulevard
Dallas, Texas 75235

Professor of surgery.

Dr. Edward Mason
(gastric by-pass)
University of Iowa Hospital
Iowa City, Iowa 52240

Professor of surgery.

Dr. Rene Menguy
Genesee Hospital
Rochester, New York 14607

*Professor of surgery,
University of Rochester.*

Dr. Frank G. Moody
(pancreas; biliary tract)
University of Utah Medical Center
50 North Medical Drive
Salt Lake City, Utah 84132

*Professor and chairman, department
of surgery.*

Dr. David Nahrwold
Department of Surgery
Hershey Medical Center
Hershey, Pennsylvania 17033

Professor of surgery.

Dr. F. Carter Nance
Tulane University Medical School
New Orleans, Louisiana 70112

Professor of surgery.

Dr. Edward P. Passaro, Jr.
(stomach)
University of California at Los
Angeles Medical Center
Los Angeles, California 90024

Professor of surgery.

Dr. Hiram Polk
Louisville University College of
Medicine
Louisville, Kentucky 40208

*Professor and chairman,
department of surgery.*

Dr. Howard Reber (pancreas)
University of Missouri Medical
Center
Columbia, Missouri 65201

Dr. Ernest Rosato
Hospital of the University of
Pennsylvania
Philadelphia, Pennsylvania 19104

Professor of surgery.

Dr. Francis Rosato (GI cancer)
Jefferson Medical College
Philadelphia, Pennsylvania 19107

*Professor and chairman,
department of surgery.*

Dr. Leonard Rosoff (stomach;
biliary tract)
University of Southern
California–Los Angeles County
Medical Center
Los Angeles, California 90033

*Professor and chairman,
department of surgery.*

Dr. H. William Scott, Jr. (gastric
by-pass; stomach; duodenum;
colon)
Vanderbilt Hospital
Nashville, Tennessee 37232

Professor of surgery.

Dr. William Silen (stomach;
duodenum; pancreas; biliary tract)
Beth Israel Hospital
Boston, Massachusetts 02215

*Professor and chairman,
department of surgery, Harvard.*

Dr. David Skinner (esophagus)
University of Chicago Hospitals
950 East 59th Street
Chicago, Illinois 60637

*Professor and chairman,
department of surgery.*

Dr. Thomas Starzl (liver
transplant; liver surgery)
University of Colorado Medical
Center
Denver, Colorado 80262

*Professor and chairman,
department of surgery. The world
leader in liver transplantation.
Also listed separately under Kidney
and Liver Transplantation.*

Dr. James C. Thompson (stomach;
colon; pancreas; duodenum;
biliary tract)
University of Texas Medical Branch
Galveston, Texas 77550

*Professor and chairman,
department of surgery.*

Dr. Kenneth W. Warren (biliary
tract)
Lahey Clinic
605 Commonwealth Avenue
Boston, Massachusetts 02215

Dr. W. Dean Warren (portal
hypertension; pancreas)
Emory Hospital
1364 Clifton Road, NE
Atlanta, Georgia 30322

*Professor and chairman,
department of surgery.*

Dr. Lawrence W. Way (stomach;
duodenum; pancreas; biliary
tract)
University of California Medical
Center
San Francisco, California 94143

Professor of surgery.

Dr. Edward Woodward (esophagus; stomach; duodenum)
University of Florida Medical School
Gainesville, Florida 32601

Professor of surgery.

Dr. Robert Zeppa (portal hypertension; pancreas)
University of Miami Medical School
Biscayne Annex
Miami, Florida 33152

Chairman, department of surgery.

Colon and Rectal Surgeons

Colon and rectal cancer is the third most common cancer and is one of the cancers increasing in incidence. Like many cancers, if it is detected early the outcome can be very favorable.

The surgeons listed in this section are noted for their outstanding work in rectal and colon surgery. Besides cancer, colon and rectal surgery involves operations for ulcerative colitis, Crohn's disease, as well as hemorrhoids (perhaps the most common procedure). Two of the surgeons on this list handle only cases of rectal and colon cancer.

COLON AND RECTAL SURGEONS

Dr. Oliver Beahrs
Mayo Clinic
Rochester, Minnesota 55901

Section head, division of surgery.

Dr. Alejandro Castro
11125 Rockville Pike
Rockville, Maryland 20852

Assistant professor of surgery, Georgetown University.

Dr. Victor W. Fazio
Cleveland Clinic
Cleveland, Ohio 44106

Dr. Donald Gallagher
3838 California Street
San Francisco, California 94118

Associate clinical professor of surgery, University of California.

Dr. J. B. Gathright, Jr.
Ochsner Clinic
New Orleans, Louisiana 70121

Associate professor of surgery, Tulane University.

Dr. Stanley Goldberg
University of Minnesota Hospitals
Minneapolis, Minnesota 55455

Director, division of colon rectal surgery.

Dr. Barton Hoexter
29 Barstow Road
Great Neck, New York 11021

Assistant clinical professor of surgery, Cornell University.

Dr. John L. Madden
123 East 69th Street
New York, New York 10021

Clinical professor of surgery, New York Medical College.

Dr. Gerald Marks
130 South Ninth Street
Philadelphia, Pennsylvania 19107

Clinical associate professor of surgery, Jefferson Medical College.

Dr. Norman D. Nigro
22811 Greater Mack
St. Clair Shores, Michigan 48080

Clinical professor of surgery, Wayne State University.

Dr. Bertram A. Portin
1616 Kensington Avenue
Buffalo, New York 14215

Associate clinical professor of surgery, division of colorectal surgery, and chairman of the division.

Dr. Stuart H. Q. Quan (cancer)
116 East 68th Street
New York, New York 10021

Chief of the rectal clinic, Roosevelt Hospital.

Dr. John H. Remington
277 Alexander Street
Rochester, New York 14607

Clinical associate professor of surgery, University of Rochester.

Dr. Eugene P. Salvati
1010 Park Avenue
Plainfield, New Jersey 07060

Associate professor of surgery, Rutgers University.

Dr. Theodore Schrock
3838 California Street
San Francisco, California 94118

Associate professor of surgery, University of California.

Dr. Norman Sohn
475 East 72nd Street
New York, New York 10021

Assistant clinical professor of surgery, New York University.

Dr. Maus W. Stearns, Jr. (cancer)
Memorial Sloan-Kettering Hospital
for Cancer and Allied Diseases
1275 York Avenue
New York, New York 10021

Head of the rectal and colon service.

Dr. G. Bruce Thow
602 West University Avenue
Urbana, Illinois 61801

Head, department of colon and rectal surgery, Carle Clinic.

Dr. M. C. Veidenheimer
Lahey Clinic
605 Commonwealth Avenue
Boston, Massachusetts 02215

Chief of colon rectal surgery.

Bone and Joint Diseases

Rheumatologists: Diseases of the Bones and Joints and Auto-Immune Diseases

Arthritis is by definition any problem of the bones and joints. As such, it is a catch-all phrase for a large number of separate bone and joint disorders such as gout, infectious arthritis, ankylosing spondylitis, and, finally, rheumatoid arthritis, which is one of the potentially most crippling forms of arthritis.

It should be borne in mind that the same basic constituents of muscle skeletal structures are formed in all organs of the body so that some diseases treated by rheumatologists have major involvement of the heart, lungs, brain, kidney, or skin as well as the joints. This is the reason that the term "connective tissue diseases" is linked to that of "arthritic diseases."

Because arthritis affects so many adults and because it is so painful, it has often been subject to much misinformation. Many "miracle cures" have been claimed for the disease, and it has been the object of considerable medical charlatanism. One rheumatologist remarked: "There is simply no miracle cure for arthritis, there is no novel therapy or drug which will make arthritis go away." Despite this, many people have sought and continue to seek and believe in the elixir that will make their pain and swelling go away. What rheumatologists prescribe instead is a conservative approach in which the disease is regarded as a chronic problem in need of long-term management. "The best doctor will try to find ways to ease the pain and discomfort," one physician said, "but he will not promise that the symptoms will be gone quickly. The best approach to arthritis, and the only approach we now have which offers real help to the patient, is to emphasize what we know works—heat, specific exercises, proper resting of the joint or joints, and, when indicated, the proper drug. The best rheumatologists will emphasize this approach as well as rehabilitation."

One rheumatologist remarked on the difficulty of convincing many patients of the value of the conservative approach: "I think too many people have become convinced that there really is a quick cure out there and we're too stuffy or out-of-date to use it. It's a serious problem we face in this field, simply convincing people that the long-term approach is the best way to alleviate the symptoms of arthritis."

Are there any signs of bad arthritis management? A heavy reliance on drugs is generally considered a sign of less than adequate care. And, warns one noted rheumatologist, if the drugs do not work, you certainly are not getting good care. Drugs are only a *part* of the total care of the arthritic patient, and by far the most commonly used and accepted drug is still aspirin. Below is a list of some of the most outstanding rheumatologists in the country. Rheumatologists generally treat the full range of bone and joint diseases, but some have special interests in certain specific disorders. These are:

Behcet's disease. This rare condition causes ulcer-type lesions in the oral and genital area.

Scleroderma. A rare but relentless systemic disorder of the connective tissue affecting the elasticity of the skin, joints, and, at times, the lungs and heart. The disease can progress rapidly, but some cases have continued twenty to thirty years.

Lupus. More formally known as Systemic Lupus Erythematosus (SLE), this connective tissue disease strikes women predominantly. It is an auto-immune disease, meaning it is caused by a malfunction of the immune system.

Gout. An inherited, metabolic disorder, it causes inflammation and severe pain but is usually treated successfully with drugs.

Amyloidosis. A rare and potentially fatal condition in which a crystalline substance settles between the cells of the body.

Polymyalgia rheumatica. A self-limiting disorder which usually strikes older women, causing pain and stiffness in the muscles and in the hips and shoulders.

Osteoarthritis. A condition usually affecting older people in which the joint cartilage degenerates; often, however, the condition does not cause serious discomfort.

Ankylosing spondylitis. Also called Marie-Strümpell disease, usually causes stiffness in the spinal joints. Considerable progress has been made in treating this condition.

Infectious arthritis. Considered the most curable form of arthritis, it is seen in any age range and in either sex. It can be dangerous, since bacteria from this disease can rapidly destroy a joint. However, the advent of penicillin has made this disease very treatable.

As noted, some of the specialists on this list have special interests in some of these arthritic disorders. Virtually everyone on this list has had extensive experience in rheumatoid arthritis because it is so common. Some rheumatologists on this list do consultive work only; others do more day-to-day patient care.

RHEUMATOLOGISTS

Dr. Roy D. Altman (osteoarthritis)
University of Miami Medical
School
Miami, Florida 33152

Associate professor of medicine.

Dr. J. Claude Bennett
University of Alabama Medical
Center
Birmingham, Alabama 35294

Professor of medicine; chief of rheumatology and immunology.

Dr. Gerson Bernhard (Behcet's syndrome)
Wisconsin Medical College
Milwaukee, Wisconsin 53226

Clinical professor of medicine.

Dr. Paul Bilka
63 South Ninth Street
Minneapolis, Minnesota 55402

Clinical professor of medicine, University of Minnesota Medical School.

Dr. Wilbur J. Blechman
909 Interama Boulevard
North Miami Beach, Florida 33162

Clinical associate professor of medicine, University of Miami Medical School.

Dr. Rodney Bluestone (ankylosing spondylitis)
Rheumatology Section
Wadsworth Veterans Administration
Hospital
Los Angeles, California 90073

Professor of medicine, University of California at Los Angeles.

Dr. Giles Bole, Jr.
Rockham Arthritis Research Unit
University of Michigan Medical
Center
Ann Arbor, Michigan 48109

Professor of internal medicine.

Dr. Kenneth Brandt (osteoarthritis)
University of Indiana Medical Center
Indianapolis, Indiana 46223

Professor of medicine; chief, arthritis division.

Dr. Jacques R. Caldwell
University of Florida Medical School
Gainesville, Florida 32610

Associate professor of medicine.

Dr. Andrei Calin (ankylosing spondylitis)
Stanford University Medical Center
Stanford, California 94305

Associate professor of medicine.

Dr. Charles L. Christian (lupus)
Hospital for Special Surgery
535 East 70th Street
New York, New York 10021

Professor of medicine; physician-in-chief, Hospital for Special Surgery.

Dr. Alan S. Cohen (amyloidosis)
Boston City Hospital
Boston, Massachusetts 02118

Professor of medicine, Boston University.

Dr. John S. Davis (lupus)
University of Virginia Medical Center
Charlottesville, Virginia 22901

Professor of internal medicine; chief, arthritis unit.

Dr. Russell Del Toro
Ashford Medical Center
San Juan, Puerto Rico 00914

Chief, department of medicine, San Juan City Hospital.

Dr. Edmund DuBois (lupus)
435 North Bedford Drive
Beverly Hills, California 90210

Clinical professor of medicine, University of Southern California Medical School.

Dr. George E. Ehrlich
(osteoarthritis; Behcet's syndrome)
Arthritis Center
Albert Einstein Medical Center
York and Tabor Roads
Philadelphia, Pennsylvania 19141

Professor of medicine and rehabilitation medicine, Temple University Medical School; director of the Arthritis Center.

Dr. Ephraim P. Engleman
University of California Medical Center
San Francisco, California 94143

Clinical professor of medicine.

Dr. James Fries
Stanford University Medical Center
Stanford, California 94305

Associate professor of medicine.

Dr. Esther Gonzales-Pares (lupus)
University Hospital
San Juan, Puerto Rico 00905

Director of rheumatic disease section.

Dr. N. Marvin Hadler
University of North Carolina Medical School
Chapel Hill, North Carolina 27514

Associate professor of medicine.

Dr. Bevra H. Hahn (lupus)
Washington University Medical
School
St. Louis, Missouri 63110

Assistant professor of medicine.

Dr. David Hamerman
Montefiore Hospital
111 East 210th Street
Bronx, New York 10467

Chairman, department of medicine.

Dr. Edward D. Harris, Jr.
Dartmouth Medical Center
Hanover, New Hampshire 03755

*Professor of medicine; chief of
connective tissue disease section.*

Dr. Louis A. Healey (polymyalgia
rheumatica)
Dr. Robert A. Willkens
Dr. Kenneth Wilske (polymyalgia
rheumatica)
University of Washington Medical
School
Seattle, Washington 98101

*All are on the medical faculty at
the University of Washington
Medical School.*

Dr. Evelyn Hess
Division of Rheumatology
Cincinnati General Hospital
Cincinnati, Ohio 45267

McDonald professor of medicine.

Dr. Gene G. Hunder (polymyalgia
rheumatica)
Mayo Clinic
Rochester, Minnesota 55901

Dr. William H. Kammerer
517 East 71st Street
New York, New York 10021

*Clinical professor of medicine,
Cornell; attending physician,
Hospital for Special Surgery.*

Dr. Thomas G. Kantor
New York University Medical
Center
550 First Avenue
New York, New York 10016

*Director, Rheumatic Disease Study
Group; chief, section on clinical
therapy.*

Dr. Stephen R. Kaplan
Roger Williams General Hospital
Providence, Rhode Island 02908

*Associate professor of medicine,
Brown University Medical School.*

Dr. E. Carwile LeRoy (scleroderma
and lupus)
171 Ashley Avenue
Charleston, South Carolina 29403

*Professor of medicine; director,
rheumatology and immunology
division, Medical University of
South Carolina College of Medicine.*

Dr. Michael D. Lockshin
Hospital for Special Surgery
535 East 70th Street
New York, New York 10021

Dr. Daniel J. McCarty, Jr. (gout)
Medical College of Wisconsin
Milwaukee, Wisconsin 53226

*Professor and chairman, department
of medicine.*

Dr. Alfonse Masi (scleroderma)
University of Illinois Medical
School
Peoria, Illinois 61606

*Professor and chairman,
department of medicine.*

Dr. Ronald P. Messner
2211 Lomas Street, NE
Albuquerque, New Mexico 87106

*Professor of medicine; chief of
arthritis program.*

Dr. Ronald W. Moskowitz
(osteoarthritis)
2073 Abington Road
Cleveland, Ohio 44106

*Professor of medicine, director of
Rheumatic Disease Unit, Case-
Western Reserve.*

Dr. David Neustadt
600 Medical Towers Building
Louisville, Kentucky 40202

*Clinical professor of medicine,
University of Louisville.*

Dr. William O'Brien
University of Virginia Medical
Center
Charlottesville, Virginia 22901

Professor of medicine.

Dr. J. D. O'Duffy
(Behcet's syndrome)
Mayo Clinic
Rochester, Minnesota 55901

Dr. Harold E. Paulus
University of California at Los
Angeles Medical Center
Los Angeles, California 90024

Professor of medicine.

Dr. Robert H. Persellin
University of Texas Medical School
San Antonio, Texas 78284

*Professor of medical microbiology;
head of the rheumatology division.*

Dr. Paulding Phelps
180 Park Avenue
Portland, Maine 04120

Private practice.

Dr. Charles H. Plotz
Downstate Medical Center
450 Clarkson Avenue
Brooklyn, New York 11203

Professor of medicine.

Dr. Gerald P. Rodnan
(scleroderma)
University of Pittsburgh Medical
School
Pittsburgh, Pennsylvania 15213

Professor of medicine.

Dr. Stanford Roth
4950 East Thomas Road
Phoenix, Arizona 85018

Private practice.

Dr. Norman Rothermich
1211 Dublin Road
Columbus, Ohio 43215

*Clinical professor of medicine, Ohio
State.*

Dr. Naomi Fox Rothfield (lupus)
University of Connecticut Health
Center
Farmington, Connecticut 06032

*Professor of rheumatology; chief,
division of rheumatic diseases.*

Dr. Emmanuel Rudd
Hospital for Special Surgery
535 East 70th Street
New York, New York 10021

Dr. Frank R. Schmid
Northwestern University Medical
School
303 East Chicago Avenue
Chicago, Illinois 60611

*Professor of medicine; chief, section
on arthritis and connective tissue
disease.*

Dr. Gordon C. Sharp (lupus)
University of Missouri Medical
School
Columbia, Missouri 65201

Professor of medicine.

Dr. John Sigler
Henry Ford Hospital
Detroit, Michigan 48202

Chief of rheumatology.

Dr. Alfred D. Steinberg (lupus)
Building 10
National Institutes of Health
Bethesda, Maryland 20014

*Senior investigator, arthritis and
rheumatology branch of National
Institutes of Health. As with all
medical care at the National
Institutes of Health, it is free; but
the patient requires a referral from
his physician, and his disorder must
fit into the research protocols
established by National Institutes
of Health. Dr. Steinberg is
specifically studying lupus.*

Dr. Mary Betty Stevens (lupus)
Good Samaritan Hospital
5601 Loch Raven Boulevard
Baltimore, Maryland 21239

*Associate professor of medicine,
Johns Hopkins.*

Dr. Charles Tourtelotte
Temple University Hospital
Philadelphia, Pennsylvania 19140

*Professor of medicine; chairman,
rheumatology section.*

Dr. Stanley Wallace (gout)
1122 Ocean Avenue
Brooklyn, New York 11230

*Professor of medicine, State
University of New York, Downstate
(Brooklyn).*

Dr. John R. Ward
University of Utah Medical Center
Salt Lake City, Utah 84132

*Professor of medicine; chief,
arthritis division.*

Dr. Howard J. Weinberger
6200 Wilshire Boulevard
Suite 1510
Los Angeles, California 90048

Dr. Thomas E. Weiss
Ochsner Clinic
New Orleans, Louisiana 70121

Professor of medicine, Tulane.

Dr. Colin Wilson, Jr.
Emory University Hospital
Atlanta, Georgia 30322

Professor of medicine.

Dr. Morris Ziff
Southwestern Medical School
Dallas, Texas 75235

Professor of internal medicine.

Dr. Jack Zuckner
522 North New Ballas Road
St. Louis, Missouri 63141

*Director, arthritis section; professor
of clinical medicine, St. Louis
University Medical School.*

Dr. Nathan Zvaifler
University Hospital
225 West Dickinson Street
San Diego, California 92103

Professor of medicine.

Orthopedic Surgeons

Orthopedic surgery has increasingly become an area both of special concentration and of subspecialization for surgeons. Because the skeletal structure extends throughout the body and because so many different problems can occur within it, subspecialization was a natural consequence. Although many orthopedic surgeons concentrate in certain areas, most of them still perform the full range of orthopedic surgery, from fracture repair to joint replacement.

There are four distinct subspecialties of orthopedic surgery which require and have their own separate listings in this book. These are: hand surgery, sports medicine, pediatric orthopedics, and limb replantation surgery.

However, within general orthopedic surgery there are also special interests practiced by orthopedists. They are:

1. *Joint replacement.* This involves total replacement of joints using metal and plastic parts. The hip and knee are the joints most commonly replaced. Replacement of elbow, shoulder, and ankle is still in the experimental stage. The most frequent causes of joint replacement surgery are arthritis and trauma.

2. *Fracture treatment.* Although many broken bones can be set routinely in hospital emergency rooms, the more complex repairs require considerable expertise to allow the fractured area to heal properly and to function normally.

3. *Spine surgery.* The spine is subject to many disorders, mostly degenerative or mechanical. Surgery is very complex, involving either the cervical spine (neck) or the lumbar spine (back).

4. Bone and soft tissue tumor surgery. Although bone and soft tissue tumors are uncommon, they present very difficult problems. Tumors may appear in many parts of the skeletal system and require special surgical skills to remove them properly.

Orthopedic surgery has made extraordinary strides in the past several years. Artificial joints now make it possible to fully replace joints damaged by birth defects or injury or arthritis. Fractures and diseases that formerly rendered patients cripples are in many cases successfully repaired now. Bone tumors previously thought to be hopeless are now amenable to control by surgery, chemotherapy, and radiation.

Following is a list of outstanding orthopedic surgeons with their special interests noted, when appropriate. Separate listings for hand surgeons, sports medicine, and limb replantation follow.

ORTHOPEDIC SURGEONS

Dr. Harlan Amstutz (joint replacement)
Division of Orthopedic Surgery
University of California at Los Angeles Medical Center
Los Angeles, California 90024

Professor and chief, department of orthopedic surgery.

Dr. Henry Banks
New England Medical Center
171 Harrison Avenue
Boston, Massachusetts 02111

Professor and chairman, department of orthopedic surgery, Tufts.

Dr. Edwin G. Bovill, Jr. (bone tumors)
University of California Hospital
San Francisco, California 94143

Professor of orthopedic surgery.

Dr. Carl T. Brighton (nonunion fractures)
Hospital of the University of Pennsylvania
Philadelphia, Pennsylvania 19104

Chairman, department of orthopedic surgery. Known for his work in clinical application of electrical current to delayed or nonunion fractures. This is still in the experimental stages.

Dr. Rocco Calandruccio
(fracture treatment)
Campbell Clinic
869 Madison Avenue
Memphis, Tennessee 38103

Dr. Mack L. Clayton (joint replacement and arthritis surgery)
Denver Orthopedic Clinic
2045 Franklin Street
Denver, Colorado 80205

Associate professor of orthopedic surgery, University of Colorado.

Dr. Reginald Cooper
University of Iowa Hospital
Iowa City, Iowa 55240

Professor and chairman, department of orthopedic surgery.

Dr. Mark B. Coventry (joint replacement)
Mayo Clinic
Rochester, Minnesota 55901

Professor of orthopedic surgery, University of Minnesota.

Dr. William F. Enneking (bone tumors)
University of Florida College of Medicine
Gainesville, Florida 32601

Professor and chairman, department of orthopedic surgery.

Dr. C. McCollister Evarts (joint replacement)
University of Rochester Medical School
Rochester, New York 14627

Chairman, department of orthopedic surgery.

Dr. Albert B. Ferguson, Jr.
University of Pittsburgh
Pittsburgh, Pennsylvania 15213

David Silver professor of orthopedic surgery.

Dr. J. William Fielding (cervical and lumbar spine)
105 East 65th Street
New York, New York 10021

Clinical professor of orthopedic surgery, Columbia. Chief of orthopedics, St. Lukes Hospital.

Dr. Jorge O. Galante (joint replacement)
Rush Medical College
1753 West Congress Parkway
Chicago, Illinois 60612

Professor and chairman, department of orthopedic surgery, Rush Medical College.

Dr. William H. Harris (hip replacement)
Massachusetts General Hospital
Boston, Massachusetts 02114

Clinical professor of orthopedic surgery at Harvard.

Dr. Allan E. Inglis (arthritis surgery)
Hospital for Special Surgery
535 East 70th Street
New York, New York 10021

Clinical professor of surgery and anatomy, Cornell.

Dr. Henry J. Mankin (bone tumors)
Massachusetts General Hospital
Boston, Massachusetts 02114

Edith M. Ashley professor of orthopedic surgery at Harvard; chief of orthopedics, Massachusetts General.

Dr. Eugene R. Mindell (bone tumors)
462 Grider Avenue
Buffalo, New York 14215

Professor and head of orthopedic surgery at State University of New York at Buffalo.

Dr. William R. Murray (joint replacement)
University of California Medical Center
San Francisco, California 94143

Professor of orthopedic surgery, University of California Medical School at San Francisco.

Dr. Charles S. Neer II (shoulder repair and replacement)
161 Fort Washington Avenue
New York, New York 10032

Clinical professor of orthopedic surgery at Columbia.

Dr. Douglas J. Pritchard (bone tumors)
Mayo Clinic
200 First Street, SW
Rochester, Minnesota 55901

Instructor in orthopedic surgery at Mayo Graduate School.

Dr. Chitvanjan S. Ranawat (joint replacement)
517 East 71st Street
New York, New York 10021

Assistant clinical professor at Cornell.

Dr. Lee H. Riley, Jr. (hip and knee replacement; cervical spine)
The Johns Hopkins Hospital
Baltimore, Maryland 21205

Professor of orthopedic surgery.

Dr. Charles A. Rockwood (fracture treatment)
University of Texas Medical School
7703 Floyd Curl Drive
San Antonio, Texas 78284

Professor and chairman, division of orthopedics, University of Texas.

Dr. Richard H. Rothman (lumbar spine)
Pennsylvania Hospital
Philadelphia, Pennsylvania 19107

Associate professor of orthopedic surgery, University of Pennsylvania; chief of orthopedics, Pennsylvania Hospital.

Dr. Augusto Sarmiento (fracture treatment)
Los Angeles County–University of Southern California Medical Center
Los Angeles, California 90033

Chairman, department of orthopedics, University of Southern California.

Dr. Clement B. Sledge (joint replacement)
Peter Bent Brigham Hospital
Boston, Massachusetts 02115

Professor of orthopedic surgery at Harvard; chief orthopedic surgeon at Peter Bent Brigham Hospital.

Dr. Wayne O. Southwick (cervical spine)
Yale University School of Medicine
New Haven, Connecticut 06510

Professor and chief of orthopedic surgery at Yale.

Dr. Lee Ramsey Staub (joint replacement; arthritis; hand surgery)
Hospital for Special Surgery
535 East 70th Street
New York, New York 10021

Clinical professor of orthopedic surgery, Cornell.

Dr. Lloyd Taylor (trauma, fracture treatment)
4141 Geary Boulevard
San Francisco, California 94117

Dr. Leon Wiltse (lumbar spine)
2840 Long Beach Boulevard
Long Beach, California 90806

Dr. Philip D. Wilson, Jr. (hip replacement)
Hospital for Special Surgery
535 East 70th Street
New York, New York 10021

Professor of surgery (orthopedics) at Cornell; surgeon-in-chief at the Hospital for Special Surgery.

Hand Surgeons

The predominant types of hand surgery are for arthritis, injury repair, and correction of birth defects. All the hand surgeons on this list have extensive experience in these areas and do not further subspecialize.

Hand surgeons are orthopedic surgeons, plastic surgeons, or general surgeons who have subspecialized in hand surgery, often to the exclusion of other types of surgery. Because of the delicacy of the hand, the surgery is very exacting. Another type of surgery on the hand, replantation of amputated digits or a hand itself, is performed by some hand surgeons, and those who have experience in this area and have an active replantation service are listed in the replantation section.

HAND SURGEONS

Dr. Charles R. Ashworth
2300 Hope Street
Los Angeles, California 90007

Associate clinical professor of orthopedic surgery, University of Southern California.

Dr. Robert Beasley
New York University Medical Center
560 First Avenue
New York, New York 10016

Professor of plastic surgery.

Dr. Harry J. Buncke
39 North San Mateo Drive
San Mateo, California 94401

Assistant clinical professor of surgery at Stanford and University of California.

Dr. Robert Carroll
Columbia-Presbyterian Medical Center
630 West 168th Street
New York, New York 10032

Dr. Raymond Curtis
2947 St. Paul Street
Baltimore, Maryland 21218

Dr. James Dobyns
Mayo Clinic
Rochester, Minnesota 55901

Dr. Richard G. Eaton
428 West 59th Street
New York, New York 10019

Associate clinical professor of surgery, Columbia College of Physicians and Surgeons.

Dr. Adrian E. Flatt
University Hospitals
Iowa City, Iowa 52242

Professor of orthopedic surgery.

Dr. Avrum Froimson
11201 Shaker Boulevard
Cleveland, Ohio 44104

Assistant clinical professor of orthopedic surgery, Case-Western Reserve.

Dr. J. Leonard Goldner
Duke Medical Center
Durham, North Carolina 27710

Professor and chairman, division of orthopedic surgery.

Dr. David Green
8042 Wurzbach
San Antonio, Texas 78229

Clinical professor of orthopedics; University of Texas Medical School.

Dr. James M. Hunter
243 South Tenth
Philadelphia, Pennsylvania 19107

Associate professor of orthopedic surgery, Jefferson Medical College.

Dr. Eugene Kilgore
450 Sutter Street
San Francisco, California 94108

Clinical professor of surgery, University of California.

Dr. Harold E. Kleinert
Doctor's Office Building
250 East Liberty Street
Louisville, Kentucky 40202

Clinical professor of surgery, University of Louisville.

Dr. Robert Larsen
Professional Plaza Building
3800 Woodward
Detroit, Michigan 48201

Clinical associate professor of medicine.

Dr. Ronald Linscheid
Mayo Clinic
Rochester, Minnesota 55901

Dr. J. W. Littler
Roosevelt Hospital
425 West 59th Street
New York, New York 10019

Chief of plastic and reconstructive surgery.

Dr. Robert McCormack
Strong Memorial Hospital
Rochester, New York 14642

Professor and chairman, division of plastic surgery, University of Rochester Medical School.

Dr. Gordon McFarland, Jr.
Ochsner Clinic
New Orleans, Louisiana 70121

Dr. John W. Madden
310 North Wilmot Road
Tucson, Arizona 85711

Professor of surgery, University of Arizona.

Dr. John J. Niebauer
516 Sutter Street
San Francisco, California 94122

Clinical professor of orthopedic surgery, University of California Medical School.

Dr. George Omer
University of New Mexico Health Sciences Center
Albuquerque, New Mexico 87131

Professor and chairman, department of orthopedics; chief, division of hand surgery.

Dr. Erle Peacock, Jr.
Tulane University Medical School
New Orleans, Louisiana 70112

Professor of plastic surgery.

Dr. Daniel C. Riordan
1538 Louisiana Avenue
New Orleans, Louisiana 70115

Clinical professor of orthopedic surgery, Tulane.

Dr. Richard J. Smith
Department of Orthopedic Surgery
Massachusetts General Hospital
Boston, Massachusetts 02114

Associate clinical professor of orthopedic surgery, Harvard.

Dr. Herbert H. Stark
2300 South Hope Street
Los Angeles, California 90007

Professor of surgery, University of Southern California Medical School.

Dr. James W. Strickland
8402 Harcourt Road
Indianapolis, Indiana 46260

Director of hand service, University of Indiana Medical Center.

Dr. William Stromberg
707 Fairbanks Court
Chicago, Illinois 60611

Assistant professor of orthopedic surgery, Northwestern University.

Dr. Alfred B. Swanson
1900 East Wealthy Street
Grand Rapids, Michigan 49506

Clinical professor of surgery, Michigan State University College of Human Medicine.

Dr. Paul M. Weeks
Washington University Medical School
St. Louis, Missouri 63110

Professor of plastic surgery.

Sports Medicine Specialists

One of the most recent medical specialties is sports medicine. The recent resurgence of interest in exercise has created a heavy demand in this field since so many people injure themselves in their pursuit of physical fitness. Most sports medicine specialists are orthopedic surgeons who have concentrated their efforts on knees, elbows, and shoulders, the most vulnerable areas for both professional and weekend athletes. Sports medicine specialists are also placing heavy emphasis on preventive measures, such as strengthening exercises and proper equipment to minimize the possibility of sports-related injuries. Sports medicine has also had an impact on rules and playing conditions. The crackback block is now prohibited in football because research revealed it caused too many knee injuries. Potentially fatal heat strokes have been reduced because of studies that showed the players' need for water when the temperature and humidity reached a certain point during football practice. Studies on shoes and playing surfaces have also resulted in improved equipment for various sports activities. Listed below are some of the best in this new field and their special interests. The vast majority of sports medicine specialists subspecialize in knee repair.

SPORTS MEDICINE SPECIALISTS

Dr. Frederick L. Behling (general)
Palo Alto Medical Clinic
300 Homer Avenue
Palo Alto, California 94301

Dr. John A. Bergfeld (knee)
Cleveland Clinic
Cleveland, Ohio 44106

Dr. William G. Clancy, Jr.
Sports Medicine Section
University of Wisconsin Hospitals
1300 University Avenue
Madison, Wisconsin 53706

Head of the section on sports medicine.

Dr. Kenneth E. DeHaven (knee)
University of Rochester
Medical School
Rochester, New York 14642

Dr. James Garrick (rehabilitation and injury prevention)
Virginia Park Medical Building
333 East Virginia Avenue
Phoenix, Arizona 85004

Dr. Jack Hughston (knee)
Hughston Orthopedic Clinic
105 Physicians Building
Columbus, Georgia 31901

Dr. Douglas W. Jackson (knee)
2840 Long Beach Boulevard
Suite 410
Long Beach, California 90806

Dr. Stanley James
(running injuries)
Orthopedic and Fracture Clinic
750 East 11th Avenue
Eugene, Oregon 97401

Dr. Frank Jobe
(elbow and arm repair)
575 East Hardy
Inglewood, California 90301

Dr. Robert Kerlan
(elbow and arm surgery)
575 East Hardy
Inglewood, California 90301

Dr. Robert L. Larson
(shoulder and arm repair)
Orthopedic and Fracture Clinic
750 East 11th Avenue
Eugene, Oregon 97401

Dr. Frank C. McCue III
(knee and hand repair)
University of Virginia Hospital
Charlottesville, Virginia 22904

Dr. John L. Marshall (knee)
Hospital for Special Surgery
535 East 70th Street
New York, New York 10021

Dr. James A. Nicholas (knee)
Institute of Sports Medicine
130 East 77th Street
New York, New York 10021

Dr. Robert Nirschl
(tennis elbow, shoulder repair)
3801 North Fairfax Drive
Arlington, Virginia 22203

Dr. Gerald A. O'Connor
Department of Orthopedic Surgery
University of Michigan
Medical Center
Ann Arbor, Michigan 48104

General sports medicine.

Dr. Don H. O'Donoghue (knee)
St. Anthony's Hospital
1000 North Lee Street
Oklahoma City, Oklahoma 73102

Considered the father of sports medicine. Still very active.

Dr. Donald B. Slocum (knee)
Orthopedic and Fracture Clinic
750 East 11th Avenue
Eugene, Oregon 97401

Dr. Joseph Torg (knee)
Sports Medicine Center
Hospital of the University of
Pennsylvania
Philadelphia, Pennsylvania 19104

Dr. Hugh S. Tullos
(elbow and shoulder repair)
Department of Orthopedic Surgery
Methodist Memorial Hospital
6516 Bertner Boulevard
Houston, Texas 77030

Chief of orthopedic surgery at Methodist.

Dr. Bertram Zarins (knee)
Massachusetts General Hospital
Boston, Massachusetts 02114

Limb and Digit Replantation Specialists

Contrary to widespread belief that severed parts of the body must be reattached immediately, they can be replanted several hours after they have been severed, if properly cared for. An arm or leg can be replanted up to six or eight hours after it has been severed; a finger can wait longer to be replanted if refrigerated. The fact that this time lag exists can allow injured people to be transported to major replantation centers.

There are a number of steps that should be taken immediately, according to replantation specialists.

1. Collect all parts of the severed section. If you are within fifteen minutes or less of a hospital emergency room, go there immediately. Most emergency room personnel and paramedic personnel have been trained to deal with accidental amputations.

2. If you are a substantial distance from an emergency room, collect the severed section, wrap it in a clean towel or cloth, place it in a plastic bag, and put it in iced water. *Never* dry ice. Putting ice and water in a bucket will do fine in an emergency. Do *not* freeze the severed part. A temperature of 4°C (your refrigerator's temperature) is ideal for the preservation of the severed section.

3. It goes without saying that the injured person must be attended. The bleeding must be stopped or slowed as much as possible. Pressure over the wound with a clean towel or dressing is safer and as effective as a tourniquet.

It should be noted that not everything that is severed can be reattached and, in the words of one replantation surgeon, not everything should be. Sometimes the severed part is too mutilated to be successfully replanted. However, when the severed part is deemed acceptable for replantation, the major replantation centers are reporting a better than 90 percent success rate. Replantation specialists also agree on one principle: If a part of the body is severed and if it is at all possible, the best procedure is to get to a major replantation center. If time is too short or if transportation is impossible, then an effort should be made to get to a major medical center.

The replantation centers have a 24-hour-a-day service. Some have helicopter pads for emergency transportation, and in many states police helicopters take accident victims to the major centers. If you are in need of a replant, police should be contacted. When the emergency is underway, the replantation team is assembled and the replantation begins.

Although fingers are the most commonly severed parts of the body, arms, legs, toes, ears, hands, scalps, and penises have also been successfully replanted. The operating microscope, often used by neurosurgeons, has revolutionized replantation. Because the operating microscope magnifies the field of operation so enormously, it permits the reattachment of vessels and nerves down to 0.5 millimeters in diameter. Also, the fact that the operating microscope is very expensive and not available at many smaller hospitals is another reason to get to a major replantation center or at least a major medical center for your replantation.

As in all types of difficult surgery, experience greatly increases the skill and success rate of the surgical team. The centers and individuals listed here are recognized as the most experienced in replantation. The surgeons listed come from many specialties, including plastic surgery, hand surgery, orthopedic surgery, and general surgery. The first name on each team at each of the centers is the chief. In cases where only one doctor is listed for a center, the replantation service is covered by the hospital staff on a 24-hour basis. It should also be noted that not every member of the team operates in every case.

Because of the emergency nature of replantation, the main telephone numbers of hospitals where the replantation teams operate are listed. *In an emergency, call the number of the doctor first.* If the doctor is unreachable, call the hospital. In some cases, the surgeons do not have numbers separate from the medical center, so both they and the center are reachable at the same number. Also, the centers are listed regionally. Remember, alert the doctor or hospital or both *before* you come to them. Medical emergency personnel should guide you.

LIMB AND DIGIT REPLANTATION SPECIALISTS
EAST

Boston, Massachusetts
Massachusetts General Hospital
(617) 726–2000

Dr. Ronald Malt
Dr. James May
Dr. Richard J. Smith
(617) 726–2821 or 3580

Bronx, New York
Montefiore Hospital
(212) 920–4141

Dr. Berish Strauch
Dr. Avron Danillier
Dr. Leonard Sharzer
(212) 920–5551

Philadelphia, Pennsylvania
Thomas Jefferson University
Hospital
(215) 928–6000

Dr. James Hunter
Dr. Lawrence Schneider
(215) 629–0980

Baltimore, Maryland
Union Memorial Hospital
(301) 235–7200

Dr. Raymond Curtis
Dr. Gaylord Clark
Dr. Frederik Hanson
Dr. E. F. Shaw Wilgis
(301) 235–1603

SOUTH

Durham, North Carolina
Duke Medical Center
(919) 684–8111

Dr. James Urbaniak
Dr. Donald Bright
(Same as medical center)

Memphis, Tennessee
Baptist Hospital
(901) 522–5252

Dr. Philip Wright
Dr. Greer Richardson
(901) 525–2531

Atlanta, Georgia
Emory University Hospital
(404) 329–7201

Dr. M. J. Jurkiewicz
Dr. Foad Nahai
(404) 321–0111

Louisville, Kentucky
Jewish Hospital
(502) 587–4011

Dr. Harold Kleinert
Dr. Erdagan Atasoy
Dr. Joseph Kutz
Dr. Graham Lister
(502) 582–1634

Miami, Florida
Mercy Hospital
(305) 854–4400

Dr. Phillip George
(305) 856–3540

Gainesville, Florida
University of Florida Medical Center
(904) 392–3261

Dr. Hal G. Bingham
Dr. H. Hollis Caffee
(904) 392–3711

MIDWEST

Rochester, Minnesota
Mayo Clinic
(507) 284–2511

Dr. William Cooney
Dr. James Dobyns
Dr. Ronald Linscheid
Dr. Michael Wood
(507) 284–2994

Chicago, Illincis
Rush–Presbyterian–St. Luke's
Medical Center
(312) 942–5000

Dr. Robert Schenck
(312) 738–3426

Chicago, Illinois
University of Illinois Hospital
(312) 996–7000

Dr. Boonmee Chunprapaph
(312) 996–7161

Indianapolis, Indiana
St. Vincent's Hospital
(317) 871–2345

Dr. James B. Steichen
Dr. James Strickland
Dr. William B. Kleinman
(317) 257–9105

Springfield, Illinois
Memorial Medical Center
(217) 788–3000

St. John's Hospital
(217) 544–6464

Dr. Elvin Zook
Dr. Allen Van Beek
(217) 782–6080

Doctors Zook and Van Beek
perform replantations at both
hospitals.

WEST

Houston, Texas
Methodist Hospital
(713) 790–3311

Dr. Melvin Spira
Dr. Joseph Agirs
(713) 790–4540

Salt Lake City, Utah
University of Utah Medical Center
(801) 581–2121

Dr. Clifford Snyder
Dr. Earl Z. Browne, Jr.
(801) 582–0952

PACIFIC COAST

San Francisco, California
Ralph K. Davies Medical
Center–Franklin Hospital
(415) 565–6779

Dr. Harry Buncke
(415) 342–8989
(San Mateo, California)

Dr. Michael Brownstein
(415) 861–8040

Dr. Elliott Rose
(415) 692–3228

Dr. Thomas Noris
(415) 653–2631

Dr. Thomas Gant
(415) 821–8804

Oakland, California
Samuel Merritt Hospital
(415) 655–4000

Dr. Jack Tupper
(415) 893–9589

Los Angeles, California
University of California at Los
Angeles Medical Center
(213) 825–9111

Dr. Malcolm Lasavoy
(Same as medical center)

Orange, California
University of California at
Irvine Medical Center
(714) 634–6011

Dr. David W. Furnas
Dr. Arthur Salabian
Dr. Bruce H. Achauer
(714) 997–4300

CANADA

Montreal, Quebec
Royal Victoria Hospital
(514) 842–1231

Dr. Roland Daniel
Dr. Julia Terzis
(Same as hospital)

London, Ontario
Victoria Hospital
(519) 432–5241

Dr. Robert McFarland
Dr. Lawrence N. Hurst
(Same as hospital)

Toronto, Ontario
Toronto General Hospital
(416) 595–3111

Dr. Ralph Manktelow
Dr. Ronald Zuker
Dr. Nancy McKee
(416) 675–1741

Diseases of the Skin

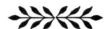

Skin Disease Specialists

Although most dermatologists treat a wide range of skin diseases, most of them also have special interests in certain skin problems.* The following are the major categories of skin diseases in which dermatologists have special nterests.

Psoriasis. Some six million Americans are afflicted with this disease. In some cases, the disease remains localized, but in others it can spread to much of the body, causing extreme discomfort. Recently new techniques involving a combination of drug and ultraviolet therapy have had remarkable results in clearing up the symptoms, but not curing this skin disease.

Skin cancer. The most curable of all cancers, skin cancers can usually be halted and surgically removed when caught early. Repeated overexposure to the sun is a major cause of this disease, dermatologists agree, and like psoriasis treatment, many new techniques have been developed in recent years that often make skin cancer surgery in the hands of an expert a minor procedure. The Mohs chemosurgery fixed tissue technique is one of the newest surgical approaches. Skin cancer should not be confused with melanoma, a skin cancer derived from pigment producing cells which can spread elsewhere in the body. Melanoma experts are listed in the cancer section.

* Pediatric dermatologists are listed in Part III, under the section "Diseases of the Skin."

Dermatopathology. Specialists in this area analyze skin tissue to determine the nature of the lesion. As one dermatologist remarked, "You don't want to have half your face taken off because of something benign, and on the other hand you don't want something ignored if it is malignant." Dermatopathologists do much of their work in laboratories, but they do see patients on a consultative basis.

Light-sensitivity. Also called photosensitivity, this disorder causes many people skin problems when exposed to sunlight. There are treatments which minimize the problems of sun sensitivity and allow people to lead a more normal life.

Immunology. Also called immuno-dermatology, this specialty involves problems with the immune response system which causes a number of skin disorders. Lupus of the skin, recurrent skin infections, allergies, bullous skin diseases (which cause skin blistering), blood vessel inflammation in the skin are some of the problems caused by immune system disorders.

Contact dermatitis and eczema. Contact dermatitis is an inflammation of the skin caused when it comes into contact with different types of chemical toxins. Eczema is also an inflammation of the skin. These similar skin problems can be treated routinely in many cases but, as in psoriasis, at times the diseased area of the skin is extensive and requires serious medical attention.

Hair problems. Excessive hair growth or hair loss is a special interest of some dermatologists. Excessive hair growth for women is also an area in which reproductive endocrinologists and general endocrinologists investigate. Unusual hair loss—other than normal balding (often due to a heredity factor)—can be caused by a number of organic problems, some of which can be controlled or reversed.

Hair transplants. Some noted dermatologists do cosmetic hair transplants in which hair "plugs" are placed in the scalp and replace lost hair.

Fungus infections. Some skin problems are caused by fungus infections and must be treated differently from other types of skin infections. This area is a special interest of some dermatologists.

Pigmentation diseases. Skin pigmentation problems, which may cause severe skin blotching, are a special interest of some dermatologists.

Acne. Although usually associated with the teen-age years, this disorder can persist much later into life and at times, because of its seriousness, require specialized treatment with drugs and external skin treatments.

Dermabrasion. Also called *cosmetic skin surgery*, this is a technique by which superficial facial scarring is removed by a brushing technique.

General dermatology. Most dermatologists listed here do general dermatology, which encompasses the wide variety of skin disorders; they are so listed, and most of those listed with special interests also treat other dermatologic problems besides those for which they are especially noted.

DERMATOLOGISTS

Dr. Bernard A. Ackerman
(dermatopathology)
New York University
Medical Center
562 First Avenue
New York, New York 10016

*Professor, departments of
dermatology and pathology.*

Dr. Wilma Bergfeld
(hair problems)
Cleveland Clinic
Cleveland, Ohio 44106

Dr. David Bickers
(light-sensitivity)
University Hospitals
Cleveland, Ohio 44106

*Professor of dermatology,
Case-Western Reserve.*

Dr. Donald Birmingham
(contact dermatitis)
Wayne State University
Medical School
Detroit, Michigan 48201

Professor of dermatology.

Dr. Harvey Blank
(infectious skin diseases)
University of Miami Medical School
Miami, Florida 33152

*Professor and chairman, department
of dermatology.*

Dr. Irwin M. Braverman (psoriasis)
Yale University Medical School
New Haven, Connecticut 06510

Professor of dermatology.

Dr. Thomas K. Burnham
(immunology)
Henry Ford Hospital
Detroit, Michigan 48202

*Clinical associate professor of
dermatology, University of
Michigan.*

Dr. William A. Caro
(general dermatology)
Northwestern University
Medical School
303 East Chicago Avenue
Chicago, Illinois 60611

Professor of dermatology.

Dr. Wallace Clark
(dermatopathology)
Temple University Medical School
Philadelphia, Pennsylvania 19140

*Professor of dermatology.
Known for his expertise in
melanoma analysis.*

Dr. William Clendenning
(general dermatology)
Mary Hitchcock Memorial Hospital
Hanover, New Hampshire 03755

*Clinical professor of medicine
(dermatology).*

Dr. David L. Cram (psoriasis)
University of California
Medical Center
San Francisco, California 94143

Chief of the dermatology clinic; associate professor of medicine.

Dr. Luis Diaz (immunology)
University of Michigan
Medical Center
Ann Arbor, Michigan 48109

Associate professor of dermatology.

Dr. John Epstein
(skin cancer; light-sensitivity)
450 Sutter Street
San Francisco, California 94108

Clinical professor of dermatology, University of California.

Dr. Mark Allen Everett
(skin cancer)
University of Oklahoma
Health Sciences Center
Oklahoma City, Oklahoma 73190

Professor and chairman, department of dermatology.

Dr. Eugene M. Farber (psoriasis)
Stanford University Medical Center
Stanford, California 94305

Professor and chairman, department of dermatology.

Dr. Alex Fisher
(contact dermatitis; eczema)
923 Fifth Avenue
New York, New York 10021

Dr. Thomas Fitzpatrick (psoriasis)
Massachusetts General Hospital
Boston, Massachusetts 02114

The Edmund Wigglesworth professor of dermatology, Harvard.

Dr. Robert G. Freeman
(dermatopathology)
8350 North Central Expressway
Dallas, Texas 75206

Clinical professor of pathology and dermatology, Southwestern Medical School.

Dr. James Gilliam (immunology)
Southwestern Medical School
Dallas, Texas 75235

Associate professor of dermatology.

Dr. Robert W. Goltz
(dermatopathology)
University of Minnesota Hospital
Minneapolis, Minnesota 55455

Professor and chairman, department of dermatology.

Dr. Leonard Harber
(psoriasis; light-sensitivity)
Atchley Pavilion
Columbia-Presbyterian
Medical Center
161 Fort Washington Avenue
New York, New York 10032

Professor and chairman, department of dermatology.

Dr. E. Richard Harrell
(fungus infections)
3250 Plymouth Road
Ann Arbor, Michigan 48015

Clinical professor of dermatology, Michigan.

Dr. John Haserick
(general dermatology)
Pinehurst Medical Center
Pinehurst, North Carolina 28374

Clinical professor of dermatology, Duke.

Dr. J. Terrence Headington
(dermatopathology)
University of Michigan
Medical Center
Ann Arbor, Michigan 48109

*Professor of pathology and
dermatology.*

Dr. James H. Herndon, Jr.
(general dermatology)
Southwestern Medical School
Dallas, Texas 75235

Associate professor of dermatology.

Dr. Harry J. Hurley
(general dermatology)
39 Copley Road
Upper Darby, Pennsylvania 19082

*Professor of dermatology, University
of Pennsylvania.*

Dr. G. Thomas Jansen
(dermabrasion)
University of Arkansas
Medical Center
Little Rock, Arkansas 72205

*Professor and chairman, department
of dermatology.*

Dr. Michael T. Jarratt
(psoriasis; light-sensitivity)
6655 Travis Street
Houston, Texas 77030

*Associate professor of dermatology,
Baylor.*

Dr. Wayne C. Johnson
(dermatopathology)
Skin and Cancer Hospital
3322 North Broad Street
Philadelphia, Pennsylvania 19140

*Professor of dermatology, Temple
Medical School.*

Dr. Henry W. Jolly, Jr.
(general dermatology)
Louisiana State University
Medical School
Baton Rouge, Louisiana 70803

*Clinical professor and head,
department of dermatology.*

Dr. Henry Jones
(fungus infections)
Emory University Hospitals
Atlanta, Georgia 30308

Professor of dermatology.

Dr. Robert Jordan (immunology)
Medical College of Wisconsin
Milwaukee, Wisconsin 53233

*Professor and chairman, section on
dermatology. A special interest in
lupus.*

Dr. William P. Jordan, Jr.
(contact dermatitis; eczema)
Medical College of Virginia
Richmond, Virginia 23298

Associate professor of dermatology.

Dr. Steven I. Katz (immunology)
Room 12N238
Building 10
National Cancer Institute
National Institutes of Health
Bethesda, Maryland 20014

*Like all National Institutes of
Health patient care, there is no
fee. However, anyone wishing
to go to the National Institutes
of Health for medical care must
have a referral from his or her
physician and must have a disease
which fits into the National
Institutes of Health research
protocols.*

Dr. Robert E. Kellum
(general dermatology)
The Mason Clinic
1118 Ninth Avenue
Seattle, Washington 98101

Dr. John A. Kenny, Jr.
(pigmentation diseases)
Howard University Hospital
Washington, District of Columbia
20006

*Professor and chairman, department
of dermatology. Dr. Kenny has
specialized in pigmentation
diseases of blacks.*

Dr. W. R. Knowles
(hair transplants)
1506 Memorial Professional
Building
Houston, Texas 77002

*Clinical instructor in dermatology at
Baylor and the University of Texas.*

Dr. John Knox
(skin cancer and dermatopathology)
Baylor College of Medicine
Houston, Texas 77025

*Professor and chairman, department
of dermatology.*

Dr. Alfred W. Kopf (skin cancer)
New York University Skin and
Cancer Hospital
566 First Avenue
New York, New York 10016

*Professor of dermatology,
New York University.*

Dr. Edward Krull (skin surgery)
Henry Ford Hospital
2799 West Grand Boulevard
Detroit, Michigan 48202

*Chairman, department of
dermatology.*

Dr. Aaron B. Lerner
(pigmentation diseases)
Yale University Medical School
New Haven, Connecticut 06510

*Director, department of
dermatology.*

Dr. Walter Lever
(dermatopathology)
280 Washington Street
Suite 307
Brighton, Massachusetts 02135

*Professor emeritus at Tufts. An
elder statesman in this field,
highly respected and still active.*

Dr. Allan L. Lorincz
(general dermatology)
University of Chicago Hospitals
950 East 59th Street
Chicago, Illinois 60637

Professor of dermatology.

Dr. Peter J. Lynch
(general dermatology)
University of Arizona
Medical Center
Tucson, Arizona 85724

*Professor of internal medicine
(dermatology); chief of the
division of dermatology.*

Dr. Howard Maibach
(contact dermatitis; cosmetic injury)
University of California
Medical Center
San Francisco, California 94143

Professor of dermatology.

Dr. Beno Michel (immunology)
University Hospitals
Cleveland, Ohio 44106

*Associate clinical professor of
dermatology, Case-Western
Reserve.*

Dr. Martin C. Mihn, Jr.
(dermatopathology)
Department of Pathology
Massachusetts General Hospital
Boston, Massachusetts 02114

Chief of dermatopathology service; professor of pathology; assistant professor of dermatology.

Dr. Frederick Mohs (skin cancer)
University Hospitals
1300 University Avenue
Madison, Wisconsin 53706

Clinical professor of surgery, University of Wisconsin. Chemosurgery fixed tissue technique, also called Mohs excision, was developed by Dr. Mohs for treatment of skin cancer.

Dr. Samuel Moschella
(general dermatology)
Lahey Clinic
605 Commonwealth Avenue
Boston, Massachusetts 02215

Also a special interest in skin cancer.

Dr. John Parrish
(psoriasis; light-sensitivity)
Massachusetts General Hospital
Boston, Massachusetts 02114

Dr. Harold Perry
(general dermatology)
Mayo Clinic
Rochester, Minnesota 55901

Director of dermatology.

Dr. Peter E. Pochi (acne)
720 Harrison Avenue
Boston, Massachusetts 02118

Professor of dermatology, Boston University Medical School.

Dr. Thomas Provost (immunology)
The Johns Hopkins Hospital
Baltimore, Maryland 21205

Associate professor of dermatology.

Dr. Rees B. Rees
(general dermatology)
450 Sutter Street
San Francisco, California 94108

Clinical professor of dermatology, University of California.

Dr. Perry Robbins (skin cancer)
New York University
Medical Center
562 First Avenue
New York, New York 10016

Professor of dermatology.

Dr. Henry H. Roenigk, Jr.
(psoriasis)
Northwestern University
Medical School
303 East Chicago Avenue
Chicago, Illinois 60611

Professor of dermatology.

Dr. W. Mitchell Sams, Jr.
(light-sensitivity)
University of North Carolina
Memorial Hospital
Chapel Hill, North Carolina 27514

Professor of dermatology.

Dr. Gordon C. Sauer
6400 Prospect Avenue
Kansas City, Missouri 64132

Clinical professor of medicine (dermatology), University of Kansas.

Dr. Walter B. Shelley
(general dermatology)
Hospital of the University of
Pennsylvania
Philadelphia, Pennsylvania 19104

*Chairman, department of
dermatology.*

Dr. Edgar B. Smith
(fungus infections)
University of Texas Medical Branch
Galveston, Texas 77550

*Chairman, department of
dermatology.*

Dr. Richard Stoughton (psoriasis)
University Hospital
225 West Dickinson Street
San Diego, California 92103

*Professor of medicine, University of
California.*

Dr. John S. Strauss (acne)
University of Iowa Hospitals
Iowa City, Iowa 52242

*Professor and chairman, department
of dermatology.*

Dr. William B. Taylor II
(skin cancer)
University of Michigan
Medical Center
Ann Arbor, Michigan 48109

Professor of dermatology.

Dr. Theodore A. Tromovitch
(skin cancer; hair transplants;
dermabrasion)
350 Parnassus Avenue
San Francisco, California 94117

*Associate clinical professor of
dermatology, University of
California.*

Dr. Denny Tuffanelli
(immunology)
450 Sutter Street
San Francisco, California 94108

*Associate clinical professor of
dermatology, University of
California.*

Dr. Eugene Van Scott
(skin cancer; psoriasis)
Skin and Cancer Hospital
3322 North Broad Street
Philadelphia, Pennsylvania 19140

Professor of dermatology, Temple.

Dr. John J. Voohrees
(psoriasis)
Department of Dermatology
University of Michigan
Medical Center
Ann Arbor, Michigan 48109

*Professor and chairman, department
of dermatology.*

Dr. Gerald D. Weinstein
(psoriasis; skin cancer)
Department of Dermatology
University of Miami Medical School
Biscayne Annex
Miami, Florida 33152

Professor of dermatology.

Dr. William Weston (immunology)
University of Colorado
Medical Center
Denver, Colorado 80220

*Chairman, department of
dermatology.*

Dr. Clayton Wheeler (infections)
North Carolina University Memorial
Hospital
Chapel Hill, North Carolina 27514

*Professor, and chairman of
dermatology department.*

Dr. Isaac Willis
(light-sensitivity)
Buckhead Medical Buildings
3312 Piedmont Road, NE
Atlanta, Georgia 30305

*Associate professor of medicine,
Emory University.*

Kidney and Urinary Disorders

Kidney Disease

Because the medical management of kidney patients on dialysis is so expensive, a special act of Congress was passed which pays all medical expenses for dialysis. However, the fact that the government reimburses the cost of medical care—thereby guaranteeing payment—has led to abuses in this field. Several kidney specialists noted the recent appearance of what they called "storefront" kidney dialysis units which are profit-making ventures. As one kidney specialist noted, "These operations have a proprietary interest in keeping the patient on dialysis and in not making them available for possible transplants, simply because if they are transplanted, they leave the dialysis unit." These new dialysis units are especially prevalent in the Midwest and in parts of California, they said.

What are signals to be wary of if you are a kidney patient and uncertain whether you are getting the best of care?

1. It is strong evidence of bad kidney patient care if you are confused about your diagnosis or the long-term plan for your care despite your efforts to find out.

2. If you are under the age of fifty and are under dialysis for kidney disease—and without other disorders—and you are without an option for kidney transplantation, you should, says one kidney specialist, view your care as "suspect."

3. If you are on dialysis and do not thrive and find yourself unable to resume your normal work or home responsibilities, further consultation is appropriate.

At present there are 42,000 people on kidney dialysis in this country and less than 10 percent of them will get a kidney transplant each year. Home dialysis is a relatively new innovation and has restored more normalcy to the lives of people with kidney failure. At present, dialysis requires four to six hours on the dialysis unit three times a week, for a total of twelve to eighteen hours a week. This is an enormous amount of time. There are studies now underway to determine if these six-hour sessions might be cut to three hours without impairing the well-being of the patient.

Although dialysis allows kidney patients to survive, it is not the answer to kidney failure. People on dialysis have shortened life expectancies due in large part to arteriosclerosis and high blood pressure. There is the belief that the fluid retention accelerates these cardiovascular complications.

If you can recognize the signs of an inferior kidney care specialist, what are the usual signals of a superior one? A kidney specialist remarks, "A doctor who examines urine specimens himself and doesn't leave it to a lab technician. There are many subtleties to examining a specimen that a technician would not be aware of but an experienced kidney specialist would be. If you see a kidney specialist, ask him if he looks at the urine himself. If he says no, be wary of him. I would."

There is one other factor to be aware of when under the care of a kidney specialist (nephrologist). If he recommends you for a kidney transplant procedure and gives you the name of the surgeon, ask him what the surgeon's results are. If he doesn't know or is at all vague, get another opinion. Also, see the kidney transplant list for those transplant teams that have the greatest experience and are getting the best results. All the outstanding kidney experts listed here are widely experienced in dialysis as well as in treating the full range of kidney disorders.

NEPHROLOGISTS

Dr. David S. Baldwin
20 East 68th Street
New York, New York 10021

Professor of medicine, New York University Medical School.

Dr. Christopher Blagg
Department of Medicine
University of Washington
Medical School
Seattle, Washington 98195

Associate professor of medicine.

Dr. William J. Flanigan
University of Arkansas
Medical Center
Little Rock, Arkansas 72201

Professor of medicine and director, department of dialysis and transplantation.

Dr. Richard B. Freeman
University of Rochester
Medical Center
Rochester, New York 14620

Head of renal unit; associate professor of medicine.

Dr. Eli A. Friedman
Downstate Medical Center
450 Clarkson Avenue
Brooklyn, New York 11203

Professor of medicine, State University of New York School of Medicine at Brooklyn.

Dr. Richard J. Glassock
Harbor General Hospital
1000 West Carson Street
Torrance, California 90509

Professor of medicine, University of California at Los Angeles; chief of nephrology, Harbor General.

Dr. Martin Goldberg
860 Gates Pavilion
Hospital of the University of
Pennsylvania
Philadelphia, Pennsylvania 19104

Professor of medicine, chief of renal-electrolyte division.

Dr. Phillip M. Hall
Cleveland Clinic
Cleveland, Ohio 44106

Dr. Carl Kjellstrand
University of Minnesota Hospital
Minneapolis, Minnesota 55455

Dr. Saulo Klahr
Barnes Hospital Plaza
St. Louis, Missouri 63110

Professor of medicine, Washington University.

Dr. Neil Kurtzman
University of Illinois Hospital
Box 6998
Chicago, Illinois 60680

Chief, division of nephrology.

Dr. Manuel Martinez-Maldonado
University of Puerto Rico
San Juan, Puerto Rico 00931

Dr. Shaul G. Massry
University of Southern California
School of Medicine
Los Angeles, California 90033

Chief, division of nephrology, and professor of medicine.

Dr. John P. Merrill
Peter Bent Brigham Hospital
721 Huntington Avenue
Boston, Massachusetts 02115

Professor of medicine at Harvard.

Dr. Karl D. Nolph
University of Missouri
Medical Center
Columbia, Missouri 65210

Professor of medicine; director, division of nephrology.

Dr. Victor Polluck
University of Cincinnati
Medical School
Cincinnati, Ohio 45267

Director, division of nephrology.

Dr. August R. Remmers, Jr.
University of Texas Medical Branch
Galveston, Texas 77550

Professor of internal medicine.

Dr. Roscoe R. Robinson
Duke Medical Center
Durham, North Carolina 27710

Professor of medicine; director, department of nephrology.

Dr. George E. Schreiner
Georgetown University Hospital
3800 Reservoir Road, NW
Washington, District of Columbia
20007

Professor of medicine.

Dr. Robert W. Schrier
University of Colorado
Medical Center
4200 East Ninth Avenue
Denver, Colorado 80220

Professor and chairman, department of medicine.

Dr. Belding H. Scribner
Department of Medicine
University of Washington
Seattle, Washington 98195

Professor of medicine.

Dr. Donald W. Seldin
University of Texas
Southwestern Medical School
5323 Harry Hines Boulevard
Dallas, Texas 75235

Professor of internal medicine.

Dr. Fred L. Shapiro
Hennepin County Medical Center
701 Park Avenue
Minneapolis, Minnesota 55415

Professor, department of medicine, University of Minnesota.

Dr. Wadi N. Suki
Methodist Hospital
6535 Fannin
Houston, Texas 77030

Chief, renal service, and professor of medicine at Baylor.

Dr. Samuel O. Thier
Yale University School of Medicine
333 Cedar Street
New Haven, Connecticut 06510

Professor and chairman, department of medicine.

Urologists

The urological system includes the urinary tract, kidneys and bladder, prostate gland, and male genital system. Although most urologists operate on all the parts of the urinary system, they may have special interests in specific areas, just as in many of the other specialties. In general, these special interest areas are:

1. *Kidney stones.* Sometimes they are removed by surgery, sometimes by other medical methods.

2. *Prostate surgery.* Removal of the prostate can be necessitated by malignant and nonmalignant tumors or an enlargement which, while not malignant, causes difficulty in urinating.

3. *Kidney surgery.* The removal of kidney stones and repair of blood vessels to and in the kidneys fall in this category. As a part of this, some surgeons do "kidney bench surgery," a procedure in which the kidney is removed from the body for certain disorders, operated on, and then replaced. Some vascular surgeons also have a special interest in renal artery surgery.

4. *Infertility.* Some urologists have special interest in male infertility problems.

5. *Bladder cancer.* About 9 percent of all cancers in men are bladder cancer, and a total of 26 percent of cancers in men involve the urinary system.

6. *Infections.* Most urinary infections can be treated fairly routinely, but some require specialized treatment because of their persistence or virulence.

7. *General urinary cancer.* This would include any tumors of the urologic system.

Urological surgery can be very exacting, and in the wrong hands serious, but avoidable, complications can arise. One prominent urologist commented that a substantial part of his practice involves operating on a patient a *second* time after the initial surgeon's failure to correct the problem.

The following are outstanding urologists. Where appropriate, their special interests are noted. It should also be noted that many of the outstanding urologists on this list do pediatric urology as well as adult. However, a separate pediatric urology list appears in the pediatric section.

UROLOGISTS

Dr. Samuel S. Ambrose, Jr.
Emory University Clinic
Atlanta, Georgia 30322

Professor of urology.

Dr. William H. Boyce
(stones and renal vascular surgery)
Bowman-Gray Medical School
300 Hawthorne Road
Winston-Salem, North Carolina
27103

*Professor and chairman,
urology section.*

Dr. C. Eugene Carlton
(prostate cancer)
Baylor College of Medicine
Houston, Texas 77025

*Professor and head,
division of urology.*

Dr. Abraham T. K. Cockett
University of Rochester
Medical School
Rochester, New York 14642

*Professor and chairman, department
of urology.*

Dr. Roy J. Correa, Jr.
Virginia Mason Clinic
1100 Ninth Avenue
Seattle, Washington 98111

Dr. George W. Drach (stones)
1501 North Campbell Avenue
Tucson, Arizona 85274

*Chief of urology, University of
Arizona.*

Dr. William Fair (infections)
Washington University
Medical School
St. Louis, Missouri 63110

Professor of urology.

Dr. Robert Gibbons
Virginia Mason Clinic
1100 Ninth Avenue
Seattle, Washington 98111

Dr. Ruben F. Gitties
(kidney bench surgery)
Peter Bent Brigham Hospital
Boston, Massachusetts 02115

Professor of surgery, Harvard.

Dr. James F. Glenn
Duke Medical Center
Durham, North Carolina 27710

*Professor and chairman, department
of urology, Duke.*

Dr. John T. Grayhack
(prostate cancer)
Northwestern Memorial Hospital
707 North Fairbanks Court
Chicago, Illinois 60611

*Professor and chairman, department
of urology, Northwestern.*

Dr. Donald Griffith (stones)
Baylor College of Medicine
Houston, Texas 70025

Professor of urology.

Dr. Thomas R. Hakala (cancer)
Urological Surgery
University of Pittsburgh
Pittsburgh, Pennsylvania 15261

*Professor and chief, department of
urological surgery.*

Dr. Frank Hinman, Jr.
University of California
Medical Center
San Francisco, California 94143

Professor of urology.

Dr. Joseph J. Kaufman (renal
vascular surgery and male
incontinence)
University of California at Los
Angeles Medical Center
Los Angeles, California 90024

Chief of urology.

Dr. Warren Koontz
Medical College of Virginia
Richmond, Virginia 23298

Professor and chief of urology.

Dr. John H. McGovern
114 East 72nd Street
New York, New York 10021

Professor of urology at Cornell.

Dr. J. William McRoberts
University of Kentucky
Medical School
Lexington, Kentucky 40506

Chairman, department of urology.

Dr. Richard G. Middleton
University of Utah
Salt Lake City, Utah 84132

Professor of urology.

Dr. Vincent J. O'Conor
Northwestern Medical School
303 Chicago Avenue
Chicago, Illinois 60611

*Professor of urology at
Northwestern.*

Dr. Carl Olsson (cancer)
University Hospital
75 East Newton Street
Boston, Massachusetts 02118

*Professor of urology, Boston
University Medical School.*

Dr. David F. Paulson (cancer)
Duke Medical Center
Durham, North Carolina 27710

*Associate professor of urology
at Duke.*

Dr. Paul C. Peters (prostate)
Southwestern Medical School
Dallas, Texas 75235

*Professor and chairman,
division of urology.*

Dr. Victor A. Politano
Jackson Memorial Hospital
Miami, Florida 33136

*Professor and chairman, department
of urology, University of Miami
Medical School.*

Dr. Robert K. Rhamy
Vanderbilt Medical Center
Nashville, Tennessee 37203

*Professor of urology; chairman,
urological surgical department.*

Dr. Donald G. Skinner (cancer)
University of California at Los
Angeles Medical School
Los Angeles, California 90024

Assistant professor of surgery.

Dr. Thomas A. Stamey (infections)
Stanford Medical Center
Stanford, California 94305

*Professor of surgery; chairman,
division of urology.*

Dr. Bruce H. Stewart
(male infertility)
Cleveland Clinic
Cleveland, Ohio 44106

Dr. Ralph A. Straffon
Cleveland Clinic
Cleveland, Ohio 44106

Head, department of urology.

Dr. David C. Utz (cancer)
Mayo Clinic
Rochester, Minnesota 55901

Professor of urology.

Dr. R. Keith Waterhouse
Downstate Medical Center
450 Clarkson Avenue
Brooklyn, New York 11203

*Professor and head, department
of urology.*

Dr. Patrick Walsh
The Johns Hopkins Hospital
Baltimore, Maryland 21205

Professor of surgery.

Dr. Willet F. Whitmore
(bladder cancer)
425 East 67th Street
New York, New York 10021

Professor of surgery at Cornell.

Kidney and Liver Transplantation

The first successful kidney transplant operation was performed between identical twins in Boston in 1954. Although the operation still presents a slight, immediate risk for the patient, enormous strides have been made in the use of drugs to forestall transplantation rejection during the past twenty-five years, permitting death rates of less than 5 percent a year in the best centers. Kidney transplantation is also one surgical area in which objective comparative evaluations can be made between the different surgeons and different centers which perform it. In all, about 120 medical centers in the U.S. perform kidney transplants, but only a very few perform it with substantially greater success than the rest.

Although the statistical comparison is not a guarantee that a center is doing the transplant as well as it claims—some centers and physicians have been known to exaggerate, perhaps inadvertently, their good results—the publishing of transplant results does give a more clearly objective comparison than most other areas of medicine.

If you are one of the thousands of Americans struck with kidney failure (some 50,000 Americans contract potentially fatal kidney diseases each year), what should you know about the surgeon who is suggested for your transplant surgery? The first thing you should ask the doctor who suggests the transplant surgeon is—what are his results? If the answer is vague or uncertain, look for another kidney specialist to advise you. Below is a table indicating the survival rates of the best transplant centers, both for the transplanted kidney and the patient.

SURVIVAL RATES OF SUPERIOR KIDNEY TRANSPLANT CENTERS

| | *One-Year Survival* | | *Five-Year Survival* | |
| | IMPLANTED | | IMPLANTED | |
	KIDNEY	PATIENT	KIDNEY	PATIENT
Relative as donor	>70%	>95%	>65%	>70%
Cadaver as donor	>50%	>90%	>35%	>70%

The symbol > means greater than.

If a relative of the patient is the donor, it is clear from the statistics that the survival rate of both the patient and the implanted kidney is substantially greater than if the donor is a cadaver. The reason for this is the closer the match between donor and recipient, the less drugs are needed to prevent rejection. In kidney transplant centers of lesser experience, or quality, the survival figures for both the transplanted kidney and the patient can be substantially lower.

The technical skills required to transplant kidneys are great, but by far the greater challenge for transplant teams is to keep the body from rejecting the kidney. As one kidney transplant surgeon remarked, "We're working on the trade-off between graft rejection and too much immunosuppression that lays the patient open to infection. It is a very sophisticated process that requires great expertise in both maintaining this balance and identifying any potential infections that may befall the patient. You have to know when to give up on the kidney and to remove it to save the patient's life because the cost of suppressing the rejection is going to cost the patient his life from infection. Centers with too little experience may not even recognize a patient with an infection in the first place, or they may keep the transplanted kidney in because they don't want to give up on it, and they lose the patient."

Anyone contemplating kidney transplant surgery should be aware of the risks, and his or her nephrologist (kidney specialist) should be well aware of the results the transplant center is getting before he recommends it. There are some pitfalls. For instance, if the center reports transplanted kidney survival of 60 percent for cadaver donors, but only a 70 percent patient survival rate, it is clear that what appears to be a good transplant survival rate is due to the patients being overtreated with immunosuppressant drugs and too many dying from infection.

The usual wait for a kidney transplant—if a relative does not offer one—is several weeks to several months before an appropriate kidney can be found that matches the patient's tissue type. Although the operation and the aftercare are a grueling process for patients, it is uncommon for them to refuse a second transplant attempt if the first one fails. About two thirds of the patients who have suffered a failed transplant operation make themselves available for a second. The major reasons patients want transplantation are to get off the kidney dialysis machine, which usually requires twelve to eighteen hours a week, and to increase the quality of the extended life. People with kidney failure on dialysis usually have life expectancies about equal to living related donor recipients.

Although "end-stage" kidney disease (kidney failure) is a grave disease, it does enjoy one advantage over other illnesses—it is the only illness in which all medical care is reimbursed by the federal government. This is because of a special law which was enacted in 1973 to help families pay for the enormous expenses involved in kidney disease.

In addition to kidney transplantation, liver transplantation, a newer specialty, is included here, although there is only one doctor in the United States who is noted for performing it regularly. The doctor, Thomas Starzl, who also is an exceptional kidney transplant surgeon, has performed approximately one half of the world's 360 liver transplants.

Vastly more complex and time consuming than kidney transplantation, and with a one-year survival rate of 40 percent, liver transplantation remains more in the experimental stage, even though one person has survived nearly nine years thus far. Timing is extremely critical in liver transplantation because a patient with liver failure can only survive three days (there is nothing comparable to kidney dialysis to keep him alive) and the donor livers are viable for only a few hours after removal. When a donor liver is found, it is packed in ice and flown to the hospital transplant team (Starzl's unit is in Denver) for surgery.

Those kidney transplant surgeons listed here have had the best results and have had the widest experience in kidney transplantation. There are very few centers in the country which specialize in transplantation on very young children. The age a child should be in order to be operated on by a pediatric transplant surgeon rather than an adult surgeon is not clearly defined, but generally if he or she is under the age of eight pediatric centers have the widest experience. Pediatric specialty centers for kidney transplants are listed in the pediatric section.

KIDNEY AND LIVER TRANSPLANTATION SPECIALISTS

Dr. Folkert Belzer
University of Wisconsin
Medical School
Madison, Wisconsin 53706

Professor and chairman, department of surgery.

Dr. Arnold G. Diethelm
University of Alabama
Medical School
University Station
Birmingham, Alabama 35294

Professor of surgery.

Dr. Ronald D. Guttmann
Royal Victoria Hospital
687 Pine Avenue West
Montreal, Quebec
Canada H3A 1A1

Unlike the other physicians on this list, Dr. Guttmann is not a surgeon but a kidney specialist who heads the transplant team at Royal Victoria Hospital.

Dr. H. M. Lee
Medical College of Virginia
1200 East Broad Street
Richmond, Virginia 23219

Professor of surgery.

Dr. Thomas L. Marchioro
University of Washington
Medical School
Seattle, Washington 98195

Professor of surgery.

Dr. John S. Najarian
Department of Surgery
University of Minnesota
Minneapolis, Minnesota 55455

Professor and chairman, department of surgery.

Dr. Keith Reemtsma
Columbia-Presbyterian Hospital
622 West 168th Street
New York, New York 10032

Professor and head, department of surgery.

Dr. Oscar Salvatierra
Kidney Transplant Service
University of California
San Francisco, California 94143

Professor of surgery.

Dr. Thomas E. Starzl
(liver transplantation also)
University of Colorado
Medical Center
Denver, Colorado 80262

Professor and chairman, department of surgery; Dr. Starzl is one of the few doctors in the world to attempt a liver transplant, an extremely complex surgical technique requiring up to twenty hours to complete. He is considered the world leader in liver transplantation.

Dr. G. Melville Williams
Johns Hopkins Hospital
Baltimore, Maryland 21205

Professor of surgery.

Infectious Diseases

Infectious Disease Specialists

Virtually all infectious disease experts practice in hospitals, and most of them in university-affiliated hospitals. About 750 board-certified infectious disease experts practice the specialty in the country today.

The major areas of patient care involve detecting the causes of undiagnosed fever and combating the infectious problems from immunosuppression that often develop from cancer chemotherapy. "We attempt to detect the cause of an infection through a series of very sophisticated tests," said one infectious disease specialist, "and then select the correct antibiotic and the proper dosage to use against the disease."

Like other specialists, some infectious disease experts have special interests. These are:

Fungal infections. Histoplasmosis, a potentially fatal lung infection, and *valley fever,* another potentially fatal infection that comes from the soil in the West and Southwest, are two of the more prominent and serious fungal infections. If treated properly, both can be cured.

Bacterial infections. Heart valve infections, as well as *meningitis* and *streptococcal* and *staphylococcal infections,* are included in this area.

Viral infections. Encephalitis, viral pneumonia, and *infectious hepatitis* are some of the more serious viral infections treated by infectious disease experts.

Tropical or parasitic diseases. Encephalitis (sleeping sickness), which is of parasitic rather than viral origin, is one of the most serious parasitic diseases, although many other types of disease can be contracted from parasites.

Anaerobic infections. Anaerobic infections can only grow and multiply in the absence of oxygen. Lung and brain abscesses are two of the more common types of anaerobic infection.

Rickettsial diseases. This group of diseases, named after Dr. Ricketts, who did much of the early identification of Rocky Mountain spotted fever and then died from the disease, includes some other diseases which are spread by insects, such as *typhus*, which is caused by body lice. Rocky Mountain spotted fever, once known only in the West, is now more prevalent in the East, particularly in the South.

Fever of undetermined origin. Two individuals listed are known for their expertise in long-lasting fevers (of more than one year's duration) which do not respond to treatment and whose source cannot be identified.

Listed here are some of the most outstanding infectious disease experts and, when applicable, their special disease interests.

INFECTIOUS DISEASES SPECIALISTS

Dr. John G. Bartlett
(anaerobic infections)
New England Medical Center
171 Harrison Avenue
Boston, Massachusetts 02111

Associate professor of medicine, Tufts.

Dr. Abraham I. Braude
University Hospital
225 West Dickinson Street
San Diego, California 92103

Professor of medicine, University of California at San Diego.

Dr. R. Gordon Douglas, Jr.
(viral infections)
Strong Memorial Hospital
601 Elmwood Avenue
Rochester, New York 14642

Head of infectious disease unit; professor of medicine and microbiology, University of Rochester.

Dr. Theodore C. Eickhoff
University of Colorado
Medical Center
Denver, Colorado 80220

Head, division of infectious disease; associate professor of medicine.

Dr. Joseph E. Geraci
Mayo Clinic
Rochester, Minnesota 55901

Professor of medicine, Mayo.

Dr. Lucien B. Guze
(urinary tract infections)
Harbor View General Hospital
Torrance, California 90509

*Professor of medicine, University of
California at Los Angeles.*

Dr. William L. Hewitt
University of California at Los
Angeles Medical Center
Los Angeles, California 90024

*Professor of medicine and
pharmacology.*

Dr. Edward W. Hook
(bacterial infections)
University of Virginia
Medical Center
Charlottesville, Virginia 22901

*Professor and chairman, department
of medicine. A special interest in
heart valve infections.*

Dr. George Gee Jackson
(viral infections)
University of Illinois Hospital
Box 6998
Chicago, Illinois 60680

*Chief, infectious disease section;
professor of medicine.*

Dr. Donald Kaye
Medical College of Pennsylvania
3300 Henry Avenue
Philadelphia, Pennsylvania 19129

*Professor and chairman, department
of medicine.*

Dr. Gerald Keusch
(tropical diseases)
New England Medical Center
171 Harrison Avenue
Boston, Massachusetts 02111

*Chief, division of geographic
medicine.*

Dr. A. Martin Lerner
Hutzel Hospital
Detroit, Michigan 48201

*Professor of medicine and associate
professor of microbiology and
pathology, Wayne State University;
chief of medical unit, Hutzel
Hospital.*

Dr. Gerald Medoff
(fungal infections)
Barnes Hospital Plaza
St. Louis, Missouri 63110

*Professor of medicine, Washington
University Medical School.*

Dr. Harold C. Neu
Columbia-Presbyterian
Medical Center
630 West 168th Street
New York, New York 10032

*Professor of medicine; head,
division of infectious diseases.*

Robert G. Petersdorf
(bacterial infections)
University of Washington
Medical School
Seattle, Washington 98195

*Professor and chairman, department
of medicine. A special interest in
heart valve infections and fever
of undetermined origin.*

Dr. Jack S. Remington
Stanford University Medical School
Stanford, California 94305
Professor of medicine.

Dr. Leon D. Sabath
Department of Medicine
Mayo Memorial Building
University of Minnesota Hospital
Minneapolis, Minnesota 55455
Professor of medicine; head,
infectious disease section.

Dr. Gene H. Stollerman
(bacterial infections)
City of Memphis Hospitals
Memphis, Tennessee 38103
Professor and chairman,
department of medicine,
University of Tennessee;
physician-in-chief, City of
Memphis Hospitals. A special
interest in streptococcal infections.

Dr. Morton N. Swartz
Massachusetts General Hospital
Boston, Massachusetts 02114
Massachusetts General has a
traveler's clinic for those seeking
medical attention prior to
departing to foreign countries.
Dr. Swartz is professor of medicine
at Harvard.

Dr. Marvin Turck
Harborview Medical Center
Seattle, Washington 98104
Professor of medicine,
University of Washington.

Dr. John P. Utz (fungal infections)
Georgetown University Hospital
3800 Reservoir Road
Washington, District of Columbia
20007
Professor of medicine.

Dr. Kenneth S. Warren
(tropical diseases)
University Hospitals of Cleveland
2065 Adelbert Road
Cleveland, Ohio 44106
Professor of medicine, Case-Western
Reserve.

Dr. Louis Weinstein
Peter Bent Brigham Hospital
Boston, Massachusetts 02115
Visiting professor of medicine,
Harvard.

Dr. Arthur C. White
(bacterial infections)
Indiana University Hospitals
1100 West Michigan Street
Indianapolis, Indiana 46202
Professor of medicine.

Dr. Temple W. Williams, Jr.
Methodist Hospital
6516 Bertner Boulevard
Houston, Texas 77030
Professor of internal medicine and
micro-immunology, Baylor.

Dr. Sheldon M. Wolff
(fever of unknown origin)
New England Medical Center
171 Harrison Avenue
Boston, Massachusetts 02111
Professor and chairman, department
of medicine, Tufts.

Dr. Theodore E. Woodward
(Rickettsial diseases)
University of Maryland Hospital
22 South Green Street
Baltimore, Maryland 21201
Professor and chairman, department
of medicine.

Allergies

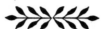

Allergists and Immunologists

Although this list names adult allergists, it should be noted that many of them see both children and adults in their practice. They all treat the full range of allergic problems, but many have special interests in certain allergic problems. These include asthma, hay fever, drug allergies (particularly to penicillin), and occupational allergies. This last category includes allergies to materials in industry as well as agriculture.

Allergy and immunology are linked into one specialty because allergic reactions are tied to an abnormal immune response in the body. Rather than creating a protective immunity, the body reacts differently and creates antibodies which do harm instead of good. Detection of the allergen is important because once known, it may be possible to avoid. If this is impossible, there are many forms of treatment that can provide relief or, in some cases, desensitization.

ALLERGISTS AND IMMUNOLOGISTS

Dr. Leonard I. Bernstein
8464 Winton Road
Cincinnati, Ohio 45231

Clinical professor of medicine, University of Cincinnati Medical Center. Co-director, Cincinnati General Hospital Allergy Clinic.

Dr. Richard S. Farr
National Jewish Hospital
3800 East Colfax Avenue
Denver, Colorado 80206

Chief, department of adult allergy and clinical immunology; professor of medicine, University of Colorado Medical School.

Dr. Kenneth P. Mathews
Allergy Clinic
University of Michigan
Medical Center
Ann Arbor, Michigan 48104

Professor of internal medicine and head of the allergy section.

Dr. Philip S. Norman
Allergy Clinic
The Good Samaritan Hospital
5601 Loch Raven Boulevard
Baltimore, Maryland 21239

Professor of medicine and chief of clinical immunology, Johns Hopkins.

Dr. Roy Patterson
222 East Superior
Chicago, Illinois 60611

Chairman, department of medicine, Northwestern University.

Dr. Charles E. Reed
504 North Walnut Street
Madison, Wisconsin 53706

Professor of medicine, University of Wisconsin. Also noted for his expertise in fungal allergies, such as "farmer's lung."

Dr. Robert E. Reisman
50 High Street
Buffalo, New York 14203

Associate clinical professor of medicine and pediatrics, State University of New York at Buffalo.

Dr. John E. Salvaggio
Tulane University Medical School
1430 Tulane Avenue
New Orleans, Louisiana 70112

Director, department of clinical immunology. Known for his expertise in occupational asthma.

Dr. Albert L. Sheffer II
110 Francis Street
Boston, Massachusetts 02215

Director, allergy clinic, Beth Israel Hospital; chief, allergy service, New England Deaconess Hospital and New England Baptist Hospital. Associate clinical professor of medicine, Harvard.

Dr. Paul P. Van Arsdel, Jr.
University of Washington
Medical Center
Seattle, Washington 98104

Professor of medicine; head, division of allergy and immunology.

Plastic Surgeons

Plastic and Reconstructive Surgeons

Although medicine is both an art and a science, plastic surgery has more art to it than any other medical specialty. Many plastic surgeons are in fact accomplished artists. "You need to be able to see how what you are doing will all come together; you need a visual imagination," one plastic surgeon said. "Experience teaches a lot," he continued, "and you need a lot of experience in plastic surgery to get truly good at it, but the one ingredient that separates the run-of-the-mill plastic surgeon from the truly gifted ones is that imagination or artistic sense."

Many procedures in plastic surgery also require a very long period of time, particularly the major reconstructive procedures. "You need experience to be able to see how things will come out in a few months from the time you do the procedure. You don't finish a reconstructive plastic surgery procedure in one day; usually there are several operations over a long period of time, and you need to be able to see how the various procedures you are doing will all come together to give you and the patient the best result. You also have to give that patient a lot of support during that long period," another plastic surgeon remarked.

There are essentially two different areas of plastic surgery. There is the major reconstructive surgery which involves the repair of injuries, burns, congenital defects, and repair of scars after cancer surgery. The second area is cosmetic plastic surgery. It must be emphasized that *all* the plastic surgeons listed here perform cosmetic surgery, such as face-lifts. However, many of those listed are also known for their work in special areas of plastic surgery for major disfigurements. These special interests are so noted. Those who do cosmetic plastic surgery either primarily or exclusively are also noted.

For clarification, here is a brief definition of some of the specialties within plastic surgery.

General reconstructive surgery. This involves the major surgical procedures to change and improve disfigurements caused by congenital defects or injury. All of the plastic surgeons listed here, expect those who do aesthetic surgery only, do general reconstruction.

Cleft lip and palate. This is a congenital birth defect in which a noticeable deformity exists in the mouth and lip. Many of the plastic surgeons on the list are noted for their repair of this problem. The procedure is often performed on very young infants, and on older patients when there is an accompanying nose deformity.

Lymphedema. Caused by a congenital absence of the lymphatic system and resulting in swelling of the legs, this condition is in some cases called elephantiasis. There is one specialist listed for this disorder.

Craniofacial reconstruction. This involves reconstruction of major —often grotesque, usually congenital—deformities or defects of the skull and face.

Breast reconstruction. This is a newer area of plastic surgery and involves the reconstruction of breasts after mastectomy.

Head and neck. Like breast reconstruction, this area involves reconstruction of scars from head and neck cancer surgery.

Reconstruction of major traumatic wounds. Such deep wounds as those from a gunshot or other severe wounds can be repaired, and new techniques have recently been developed that have greatly improved the results in this procedure.

Hand repairs. Some plastic surgeons, and some orthopedic surgeons, specialize in hand repairs. All are listed under the hand surgery section in Bone and Joint Diseases.

Mouth and jaw. This area involves the repair of mouth and jaw defects of congenital origin or due to injury or cancer surgery.

Facial reconstruction. This involves the restoring of the face and facial animation after injury or paralysis.

Genital repairs. This involves the repair of congenital defects in genitals. There is one specialist listed for this.

Aesthetic. This involves the beautifying of normal features, such as the nose, eyelids, the tightening and smoothing out of facial and neck skin, and breast reduction and lifting.

It should be noted that there is no division in plastic surgery between adult and pediatric. All plastic surgeons operate on small children for congenital defects such as cleft lip, although one surgeon is noted for his work on young children and infants. However, plastic surgeons who perform only aesthetic plastic surgery generally perform only on adults.

PLASTIC SURGEONS

Dr. Thomas J. Baker, Jr.
(aesthetic)
1501 South Miami Avenue
Miami, Florida 33129

Assistant clinical professor of plastic surgery, University of Miami Medical School.

Dr. John M. Converse
(cranial and facial reconstruction)
722 Park Avenue
New York, New York 10021

Lawrence D. Bell professor of plastic surgery, New York University Medical School.

Dr. Milton T. Edgerton
(cranial and facial reconstruction)
Department of Plastic Surgery
University of Virginia
Medical Center
Charlottesville, Virginia 22901

Professor and chairman, department of plastic surgery.

Dr. Bromley S. Freeman
(breast and facial reconstruction)
7000 Fannin
Houston, Texas 77030

Clinical professor of surgery, Baylor College of Medicine. Regarded by his peers as one of the most creative plastic surgeons. Has contributed to facial reanimation in cases of facial paralysis.

Dr. Nicholas G. Georgiade
(head and neck, jaw and breast reconstruction)
Duke University Medical Center
Durham, North Carolina 27710

Professor of plastic, maxillofacial, and oral surgery. A dentist as well as a plastic surgeon.

Dr. Dicram Goulian, Jr.
(general reconstruction)
New York Hospital–Cornell
Medical Center
525 East 68th Street
New York, New York 10021

Chairman, department of plastic surgery.

Dr. William Grabb
(cleft lip and palate)
University of Michigan
Medical Center
Ann Arbor, Michigan 48109

Professor of plastic surgery.

Dr. V. Michael Hogan
(general reconstruction)
799 Park Avenue
New York, New York 10021

*Associate professor of plastic
surgery, New York University
Medical School.*

Dr. John E. Hoops
(general reconstruction)
The Johns Hopkins Hospital
Baltimore, Maryland 21205

*Professor and head, department of
plastic surgery.*

Dr. Charles E. Horton
(repair of genital defects)
Hague Medical Center
400 West Brambleton
Norfolk, Virginia 23510

*Dr. Horton is a plastic surgeon
with an international reputation in
this subspecialty. He works with
Dr. Charles Devine, a urologist.
Also listed under pediatric urology.*

Dr. M. J. Jurkiewicz
(head and neck)
Emory Affiliated Hospitals
25 Prescott Street, NE
Atlanta, Georgia 30308

*Professor of plastic surgery;
chief, department of plastic and
reconstructive surgery, Emory.*

Dr. Thomas Krizek
(wounds; burns)
Columbia-Presbyterian
Medical Center
630 West 168th Street
New York, New York 10032

*Professor and chief, department
of plastic surgery.*

Dr. John B. Lynch
(general reconstruction)
Vanderbilt Medical Center
Nashville, Tennessee 37232

Dr. Paul R. McKissock (aesthetic
and reconstructive breast surgery)
3440 Lomita Boulevard
Torrance, California 90505

*Clinical professor of plastic surgery,
University of California at
Los Angeles.*

Dr. D. Ralph Millard
(cleft lip and palate)
1444 NW 14th Street
Miami, Florida 33125

*Clinical professor and chief,
division of plastic surgery,
University of Miami Medical
School.*

Dr. Timothy Miller
(lymphedema)
University of California at Los
Angeles Medical Center
Los Angeles, California 90024

*Professor of plastic surgery.
As noted in the introduction to
this section, lymphedema is a
lymphatic condition causing
excessive leg swelling.*

Dr. Joseph E. Murray
(head and neck)
Peter Bent Brigham Hospital
721 Huntington Avenue
Boston, Massachusetts 02115

*Professor of surgery, Harvard;
chief of plastic surgery, Peter
Bent Brigham Hospital.*

Dr. Ross Musgrave (cleft lip
and palate; congenital defects)
3600 Forbes Avenue
Pittsburgh, Pennsylvania 15213

*Professor of surgery, University
of Pittsburgh Medical School.*

Dr. Thomas D. Rees
(aesthetic)
176 East 72nd Street
New York, New York 10021

*Clinical associate professor of
surgery, New York University.*

Dr. Donald M. Serafih
(reconstruction after major
traumatic wounds)
Duke University Medical Center
Durham, North Carolina 27710

Dr. Jack H. Sheen (aesthetic
work, noses and eyelids)
9210 Sunset Boulevard
Los Angeles, California 90069

*Clinical professor of plastic
surgery, University of California
at Los Angeles.*

Dr. Melvin Spira (jaw and mouth)
Baylor College of Medicine–Texas
Medical Center
Houston, Texas 77030

*Professor and head, division of
plastic surgery, Baylor College
of Medicine.*

Dr. Richard Stark
(cleft lip and palate)
115 East 67th Street
New York, New York 10021

*Professor and chairman, department
of surgery, Columbia.*

Dr. Hugh Thomson
(pediatric only)
Hospital for Sick Children
555 University Avenue
Toronto, Ontario
Canada M5G 1X8

*Known for his repairs of all types
of defects, but especially hands of
children and infants.*

Dr. Louis Vasconez
(general reconstructive work)
University of California
Medical Center
San Francisco, California 94143

Chief, department of plastic surgery.

Dr. John E. Woods
(neck and breast reconstruction)
Mayo Graduate School of Medicine
200 First Street, SW
Rochester, Minnesota 55901

*Head, plastic surgery section.
Known for neck and breast
reconstruction following surgery.*

Dr. Harvey A. Zarem
(general reconstructive work)
Department of Plastic Surgery
University of California at
Los Angeles Medical Center
Los Angeles, California 90024

*Professor of surgery and chief,
plastic surgery division.*

Diagnostic Radiologists

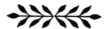

Subspecialties of Diagnostic Medicine

"Radiology," one radiologist said, "is the diagnostic hub of a hospital." It is in radiology that the diagnosis of a disease is often made, and from that diagnosis come the major decisions on how to treat it.

If a patient is already in a hospital, he or she has little choice over who takes or interprets his or her x-rays. Thus, in many circumstances knowing the outstanding radiologists does not allow you to have a consultation with them. However, in many cases prior to hospitalization there is considerable latitude in selecting a radiologist. Said one leading radiologist: "The patient and his specialist will rely heavily on the quality of the x-rays and their interpretation. However, these tests need not await referral to a clinical care specialist nor is there *any* reason why they must be performed in the specialist's hospital or clinic." This radiologist also said: "My own view is that *no* radiation is justified unless absolutely medically indicated on a case-by-case basis. Accordingly, the public should be encouraged to question their primary care physician as to the appropriateness of any diagnostic test particularly if it involves radiation, not to mention additional expense."

Because of the potential risks of radiation, these generally accepted guidelines are offered:

1. If you do not understand why the x-rays are being ordered, ask

why, and if the answer is vague, persist. If it continues to be vague, you should seek advice from another source.

2. If you are a pregnant woman, you should avoid all x-rays unless absolutely necessary, particularly x-rays of the abdomen area.

3. The time for taking x-rays of women of childbearing age should be restricted to the first fourteen days of their menstrual cycle to avoid the possibility of x-raying an early pregnancy.

4. Young adults especially should avoid any x-rays in the area of their reproductive organs.

5. Finally, if there are solid medical indications for x-ray studies, you should have them. X-rays, when interpreted by an expert who can understand their full implications, still represent one of the finest diagnostic tools in medicine.

If you are worried about your x-ray exposure, any concerned and well-trained radiologist should answer the questions you have.

All radiologists are trained in general radiology. However, many radiologists have subspecialized into different areas of diagnostic medicine. These are:

Neuroradiology. This involves x-ray studies of the brain, spine, spinal cord, and arteries leading into the brain and cord, and the use of the Computerized Tomographic Scan to diagnose brain abnormalities.

Angiography. Also called special procedures, this subspecialty involves the diagnosis of vessel and heart disease by injecting dyes into catheters placed in the vessels and heart.

GI. This involves the diagnosis of disorders of the digestive system usually by the use of barium enemas and swallows which highlight any abnormalities of the intestinal tract.

Genitourinary. This subspecialty involves the diagnosis of disorders of the urinary tract and associated structures.

Ultrasound. This is a noninvasive procedure, using sound waves, by which images can be made of various structures in the body, especially within the abdomen. It is also used in a number of areas, including cardiac problems, where it can measure many specific parts of the heart, as well as in imaging of the fetus when a problem with a pregnancy is suspected. Ultrasound does *not* emit radiation.

Bone radiology. Also called arthrography, this subspecialty is used primarily in the diagnosis of bone and joint injuries. It consists of injecting a dye into the joints to clearly outline the extent of the injury and is frequently used on athletes to determine the extent of knee and shoulder injuries, and whether or not surgery is indicated.

Chest. This involves x-rays of the heart and lungs, as well as injecting dyes into the bronchial air passages to determine the extent, if any, of blockages. It also involves the needle biopsy of lung tissue without surgery.

General diagnostic. This is just what it says—general diagnostic radiology. It can involve anything from interpreting bone fractures to lung shadows.

X-ray therapy. This involves the x-ray or radium treatment of malignancies. Outstanding x-ray therapists appear in the special section on cancer.

Pediatric radiology. Outstanding pediatric radiologists appear in the pediatric section. Outstanding pediatric x-ray therapists appear in the special section on cancer.

NEURORADIOLOGISTS

Dr. Robert E. Anderson
University of Utah Medical Center
50 North Medical Drive
Salt Lake City, Utah 84112

Associate professor of radiology.

Dr. David O. Davis
George Washington University
Medical Center
Washington, District of Columbia
20037

Professor and chairman, department of radiology.

Dr. Mokhtar H. Gado
Mallinckrodt Institute of Radiology
Washington University School
of Medicine
St. Louis, Missouri 63110

Professor of radiology.

Dr. William Hanafee
University of California
Center for Health Sciences
Los Angeles, California 90024

Professor of radiology.

Dr. Derek Harwood-Nash
Hospital for Sick Children
Toronto, Ontario
Canada M5G 1X8

Radiologist in chief. Pediatric neuroradiology.

Dr. E. Ralph Heinz
Duke University Medical Center
Durham, North Carolina 27710

Professor of radiology.

Dr. Sadek K. Hilal
Neurological Institute
710 West 168th Street
New York, New York 10032

Director of neuroradiology.

Dr. Michael S. Huckman
Presbyterian–St. Luke's Hospital
and Rush Medical College
1753 West Congress Parkway
Chicago, Illinois 60612

Professor of radiology and neurological sciences.

Dr. Bassett B. Kilgore
St. Paul's Hospital
Dallas, Texas 75235

Chief of radiology.

Dr. Irvin I. Kricheff
New York University
Medical Center
New York, New York 10016

Professor of radiology.

Dr. Thomas H. Newton
University of California
Medical Center
San Francisco, California 94143

Professor of radiology.

Dr. David Norman
University of California
Medical Center
San Francisco, California 98143

Associate professor of radiology.

Dr. D. Gordon Potts
New York Hospital–Cornell
Medical Center
New York, New York 10021

Professor of radiology.

Dr. Arthur E. Rosenbaum
Department of Radiology
University of Pittsburgh
School of Medicine
Pittsburgh, Pennsylvania 15261

Professor of radiology.

Dr. Calvin L. Rumbaugh
Peter Bent Brigham Hospital
Boston, Massachusetts 02115

*Director of neuroradiology;
professor of radiology, Harvard.*

Dr. Juan M. Taveras
Massachusetts General Hospital
Boston, Massachusetts 02114

Professor of radiology at Harvard.

Dr. Peter E. Weinberg
Northwestern Memorial Hospital
Fairbanks Court and
Superior Avenue
Chicago, Illinois 60611

Head of neuroradiology.

ANGIOGRAPHY RADIOLOGISTS

Dr. Herbert L. Abrams
Harvard Medical School
Boston, Massachusetts 02115

*Professor and chairman, department
of radiology.*

Dr. Kurt Amplatz
University of Minnesota Hospitals
Minneapolis, Minnesota 55455

Professor of radiology.

Dr. Stanley Baum
Hospital of the University of
Pennsylvania
Philadelphia, Pennsylvania 19104

*Professor and chairman, department
of radiology.*

Dr. Joseph Bookstein
University of California
Medical Center
225 West Dickinson Street
San Diego, California 92103

Dr. William Casarella
Columbia-Presbyterian
Medical Center
New York, New York 10032

Professor of radiology.

Dr. John Doppman
Building 10, Room 6S211
National Institutes of Health
Bethesda, Maryland 20014

Director, department of radiology.

Dr. Larry P. Elliott
Department of Radiology
University of Alabama
Birmingham, Alabama 35233

Professor of radiology.

Dr. Thomas Meaney
Cleveland Clinic
Cleveland, Ohio 44106

Director of radiology.

Dr. Josef Rosch
University of Orgeon Center for
Health Sciences
Portland, Oregon 97201

Professor of radiology.

GI RADIOLOGISTS

Dr. Wylie J. Dodds
Milwaukee County Hospital
Milwaukee, Wisconsin 53226

*Professor of radiology, Medical
College of Wisconsin.*

Dr. John J. Fennessy
University of Chicago Hospitals
950 East 59th Street
Chicago, Illinois 60637

*Professor and chairman, department
of radiology.*

Dr. Henry I. Goldberg
University of California
Medical Center
San Francisco, California 94143

Professor of radiology.

Dr. Igor Laufer
Hospital of the University of
Pennsylvania
Philadelphia, Pennsylvania 19104

Professor of radiology.

Dr. Ann Maria Lewicki
George Washington Hospital
Washington, District of Columbia
20037

Professor of radiology.

Dr. Alexander R. Margulis
University of California
Medical Center
San Francisco, California 94143

*Professor and chairman, department
of radiology.*

Dr. Richard Marshak
1075 Park Avenue
New York, New York 10028

*Clinical professor of radiology,
Mt. Sinai Medical School.*

Dr. Roscoe E. Miller
University of Indiana
Medical Center
Indianapolis, Indiana 46202

*Distinguished professor of
radiology.*

Dr. William B. Seaman
Columbia-Presbyterian
Medical Center
New York, New York 10032

Professor and chairman, department of radiology.

Dr. Robert J. Stanley
Washington University
Medical School
Mallinckrodt Institute of Radiology
St. Louis, Missouri 63110

Professor of radiology.

Dr. Jack Wittenberg
Massachusetts General Hospital
Boston, Massachusetts 02114

Associate professor of radiology, Harvard and Boston universities.

Dr. F. Frank Zboralske
Stanford University Medical Center
Stanford, California 94305

Director, division of radiology; professor of radiology.

GENITOURINARY RADIOLOGISTS

Dr. Joshua A. Becker
State University of New York
Downstate Medical Center
450 Clarkson Avenue
Brooklyn, New York 11203

Professor and chairman, department of radiology.

Dr. Morton A. Bosniak
New York University
School of Medicine
New York, New York 10016

Professor of radiology.

Dr. C. J. Hodson
Department of Diagnostic Radiology
Yale University School of Medicine
New Haven, Connecticut 06510

Head of GU radiology.

Dr. Bruce L. McClennan
Washington University
School of Medicine
St. Louis, Missouri 63110

Associate professor of radiology.

Dr. Alphonse Palubinskas
University of California
Medical Center
San Francisco, California 94143

Chief of GU radiology.

Dr. Lee B. Talner
University Hospital
225 West Dickinson Street
San Diego, California 92103

Associate professor of radiology.

Dr. John R. Thornbury
University of Michigan
Medical Center
Ann Arbor, Michigan 48104

Professor of radiology.

Dr. David M. Witten
University Hospital
Birmingham, Alabama 35233

Professor and chairman, department of radiology.

ULTRASOUND SPECIALISTS

Dr. Roy Filly
University of California
Medical Center
San Francisco, California 94148

Associate professor of radiology.

Dr. Barry B. Goldberg
Jefferson Medical College
Philadelphia, Pennsylvania 19107

*Professor of radiology; director,
division of diagnostic ultrasound.*

Dr. Michael L. Johnson
University of Colorado
Medical Center
Denver, Colorado 80220

Assistant professor of radiology.

Dr. Thomas L. Lawson
Medical College of Wisconsin
Milwaukee, Wisconsin 53226

Associate professor of radiology.

Dr. George R. Leopold
University of California
Medical School
San Diego, California 92103

Professor of radiology.

Dr. W. Fred Sample
University of California
Medical Center
Los Angeles, California 90024

Professor of radiology.

Dr. Roger Sanders
The Johns Hopkins Hospital
Baltimore, Maryland 21205

Professor of radiology.

Dr. Kenneth J. W. Taylor
Yale University Medical School
New Haven, Connecticut 06510

Professor of radiology.

BONE RADIOLOGISTS

Dr. Jack Edeiken
Jefferson Medical College
Philadelphia, Pennsylvania 19107

*Professor and chairman, department
of radiology.*

Dr. Robert H. Freiberger
New York Hospital–Cornell
University Medical Center
New York, New York 10021

*Professor of radiology at Cornell;
director, department of
roentgenology at the Hospital
for Special Surgery.*

Dr. Harry K. Genant
University of California
Medical Center
San Francisco, California 94143

Associate professor of radiology.

Dr. Louis A. Gilula
Mallinckrodt Institute of Radiology
St. Louis, Missouri 63110

Associate professor of radiology.

Dr. Harold G. Jacobson
Montefiore Hospital and
Medical Center
Bronx, New York 10467

*Chairman, department of radiology,
Einstein Medical School.*

Dr. William Martel
University of Michigan
Medical Center
Ann Arbor, Michigan 48104

Professor of radiology.

Dr. Tom W. Staple
Department of Radiology
Memorial Hospital Medical Center
Long Beach, California 90801

Adjunct professor of radiology,
University of California at Irvine.

CHEST RADIOLOGISTS

Dr. Kent Ellis
Columbia-Presbyterian
Medical Center
622 West 168th Street
New York, New York 10032

Professor of radiology.

Dr. John V. Forrest
6436 Avenida Cresta
La Jolla, California 92037

Associate professor of radiology,
University of California at
San Diego.

Dr. Robert G. Fraser
University of Alabama
Medical Center
Birmingham, Alabama 35223

Professor of radiology.

Dr. Paul J. Friedman
University Hospital
225 West Dickinson Street
San Diego, California 92103

Professor of radiology, University
of California.

Dr. Richard H. Greenspan
Yale University School of Medicine
333 Cedar Street
New Haven, Connecticut 06510

Professor and chairman, department
of radiology.

Dr. E. Robert Heitzman
State University of New York
Syracuse, New York 13210

Professor of radiology.

Dr. Eric N. C. Milne
Department of Radiological Sciences
University of California at Irvine
Irvine, California 92664

Professor and chairman, department
of radiology.

Dr. Charles E. Putman
Duke University Medical Center
Durham, North Carolina 27710

Professor and chairman, department
of radiology.

Dr. S. David Rockoff
George Washington University
Medical Center
Washington, District of Columbia
20037

Professor of radiology.

Dr. Stuart S. Sagel
Mallinckrodt Institute of Radiology
St. Louis, Missouri 63110

Associate professor of radiology.

GENERAL DIAGNOSTIC RADIOLOGISTS

Dr. Klaus M. Bron
Presbyterian-University Hospital
Pittsburgh, Pennsylvania 15213

Professor of radiology. Also noted for angiography.

Dr. John A. Campbell
Martin Luther King, Jr.
General Hospital
12102 Wilmington Avenue
Los Angeles, California 90059

Dr. M. Paul Capp
Arizona Medical Center
Tucson, Arizona 84724

Professor and chairman, department of radiology.

Dr. Ronald A. Castellino
Stanford University Medical Center
Stanford, California 94305

Professor of radiology.

Dr. Peter W. Cockshott
McMaster University
Medical Center
Hamilton, Ontario, Canada

Professor of radiology.

Dr. Gerald D. Dodd, Jr.
M. D. Anderson Hospital and
Tumor Institute
Houston, Texas 77025

Professor of radiology.

Dr. Theodore E. Keats
University of Virginia
Medical Center
Charlottesville, Virginia 22901

Professor and chairman, department of radiology.

Dr. Eugene C. Klatte
Indiana University Medical Center
Indianapolis, Indiana 46207

Professor and chairman, department of radiology.

Dr. Bertram Levin
University of Chicago Hospitals
Chicago, Illinois 60637

Professor of radiology.

Dr. Harry Z. Mellins
Harvard Medical School
25 Shattuck Street
Boston, Massachusetts 02115

Professor of radiology.

Dr. Lee F. Rogers
Department of Radiology
Northwestern University
Chicago, Illinois 60611

Professor and chairman, department of radiology.

Dr. Gerald T. Scanlon
Milwaukee County Hospital
Milwaukee, Wisconsin 53226

Professor of radiology, Wisconsin Medical College.

Dr. Melvyn H. Schreiber
University of Texas
Medical Branch
Galveston, Texas 77550

Professor and chairman, department of radiology.

Dr. Jerome H. Shapiro
Boston University Medical School
Boston, Massachusetts 02118

Professor and chairman, department of radiology.

Dr. Stanley S. Siegelman
Johns Hopkins Hospital
Baltimore, Maryland 21205

Professor of radiology.

Dr. Richard J. Steckel
University of California at Los
Angeles Medical Center
Los Angeles, California 90024

Professor of radiology.

Dr. Arch W. Templeton
University of Kansas
Medical Center
Kansas City, Kansas 66103

*Professor and chairman, department
of radiology.*

Dr. Joseph P. Whalen
The New York Hospital–Cornell
Medical Center
New York, New York 10021

*Professor and chairman, department
of radiology.*

Dr. Jerome F. Wiot
Cincinnati General Hospital
Cincinnati, Ohio 45267

*Professor and chairman, department
of radiology.*

Nuclear Medicine

Nuclear medicine is one of the newest diagnostic specialties in medicine. In essence, it is the diagnosis and—to a far lesser extent—the treatment of disease through radioactive isotopes.

Nuclear medicine specialists, through a process of scanning, that is, mapping the distribution within the body of injected radioactive tracer substances that measure body functions, have developed sophisticated and noninvasive methods by which to diagnose diseases. The major areas in which nuclear medicine is effective are:

Cardiology. Nuclear methods can help detect and diagnose a variety of heart disorders, especially coronary problems. They do not replace cardiac catheterization (a procedure in which a tube is inserted through a vein into the heart to measure pressures and inject x-ray contrast material), but can serve as a useful, noninvasive adjunct to it and in some cases obviate the need for catheterization.

Liver scanning. Isotope scanning of the liver and biliary system can determine the presence or absence of many different liver diseases, including tumors, cirrhosis, abscesses, and gall bladder disease.

Bone scanning. Like liver and cardiac scanning, bone scanning can determine the presence or absence of disease, including cancer, arthritis, and, to a large extent, osteomyelitis.

Cancer monitoring. Nuclear medicine techniques can determine the extent of cancer in a patient and serve as a guide to appropriate therapy.

Endocrine disorders. Although nuclear medicine is largely devoted to diagnostic and consultative medicine, there is one area of diagnosis *and* treatment and that is for endocrine disorders, mostly disorders of the thyroid gland such as hyperthyroidism and thyroid cancer. The treatment for thyroid cancer is two-fold. First, there is surgery to remove as much of the malignancy as possible. Then, a radioactive isotope is swallowed by the patient; it locates itself within the cancerous part of the thyroid, and in many cases either arrests or eradicates the cancer.

There are other uses for nuclear medicine. Nuclear medicine specialists predict that brain chemistry studies will soon be possible. These and similar studies of regional biochemistry may allow the discovery of predispositions to diseases in some people, which in turn will permit steps to be taken to arrest disease in its earliest stages.

It should be emphasized that nuclear medicine is a relatively new science and, as one nuclear medicine specialist noted, there are still few full-time nuclear medicine practitioners in the country. "To be expert at nuclear medicine you must be doing it all the time, not part-time," a nuclear medicine specialist said. "I also think it is important that the nuclear medicine specialist, not just the technicians, be there when the tests are done."

As in other medical specialties, nuclear medicine experts have special areas of interest, including nuclear cardiology and endocrinology. Those with special interests are so noted. However, except for those otherwise noted, all of the nuclear medicine specialists listed here practice the full range of diagnostic nuclear medicine.

NUCLEAR MEDICINE SPECIALISTS

Dr. James Adlestein
Peter Bent Brigham Hospital
721 Huntington Avenue
Boston, Massachusetts 02115

Professor of nuclear medicine, Harvard.

Dr. William Ashburn (cardiology)
University Hospital
225 West Dickinson Street
San Diego, California 92103

Chief of nuclear medicine division, University of California at San Diego.

Dr. David Becker (endocrine)
New York Hospital–Cornell
Medical Center
525 East 68th Street
New York, New York 10021

*Professor of medicine and
radiology; director, division
of nuclear medicine.*

Dr. William H. Beierwaltes
(endocrine)
Department of Nuclear Medicine
University of Michigan
Medical Center
Ann Arbor, Michigan 48104

*Professor of internal medicine;
director, nuclear medicine division.*

Dr. Daniel Berman (cardiology)
Cedars-Sinai Medical Center
Los Angeles, California 90048

Head of nuclear medicine.

Dr. Edward Eikman
University of South Florida
Tampa, Florida 33620

Associate professor of medicine.

Dr. Glen Hamilton (cardiology)
University of Washington
Medical School
Seattle, Washington 98101

*Dr. Hamilton practices nuclear
cardiology exclusively.*

Dr. Leonard B. Holman
Peter Bent Brigham Hospital
Boston, Massachusetts 02115

*Associate professor of radiology,
Harvard.*

Dr. Joseph P. Kriss (endocrine)
Division of Nuclear Medicine
Stanford University Medical Center
Stanford, California 94305

*Professor of nuclear medicine and
radiology; director, nuclear
medicine division.*

Dr. David E. Kuhl
Division of Nuclear Medicine
University of California at Los
Angeles Center for Health Sciences
Los Angeles, California 90024

*Professor of radiology; chief,
division of nuclear medicine.*

Dr. John G. McAfee
750 East Adams Street
Syracuse, New York 13210

*Professor of radiology and nuclear
medicine, State University of
New York at Syracuse.*

Dr. August Miale
Florida Medical Center
Department of Nuclear Medicine
500 West Oakland Park Boulevard
Lauderdale Lake, Florida 33313

*Clinical professor of nuclear
medicine, University of Miami.*

Dr. Richard Reba
George Washington
University Hospital
901 23rd Street, NW
Washington, District of Columbia
20037

*Head of nuclear medicine; professor
of radiology.*

Dr. Barry Siegel
Washington University
Medical School
St. Louis, Missouri 63110

*Director, division of nuclear
medicine.*

Dr. Richard P. Spencer
Department of Nuclear Medicine
University of Connecticut
Health Center
Farmington, Connecticut 06032

*Professor and chairman, nuclear
medicine department.*

Dr. William Strauss
Massachusetts General Hospital
Boston, Massachusetts 02114

*Associate professor of radiology,
Harvard.*

Dr. Henry N. Wagner, Jr.
Johns Hopkins Hospital
Baltimore, Maryland 21205

*Professor of medicine, radiology,
and environmental health science;
head of division of nuclear medicine.*

Dr. Barry Zaret (cardiology)
Yale–New Haven Hospital
333 Cedar Street
New Haven, Connecticut 06510

*Dr. Zaret practices nuclear
cardiology exclusively.*

PART II

Childbirth

Pediatric Genetic Counseling

Genetic counseling attempts to avoid or minimize as many inherited childhood disorders as possible. However, one of the major problems is that very few doctors know much about genetics. Genetics was only sparingly taught in medical schools before the late 1960s—thus older doctors who do not specialize in this area are likely to know little about it—and even today the genetics training in medical school is scant.

Furthermore, much of our knowledge about chromosomal (genetically transmitted) disease has been learned during the past fifteen years. Such techniques as prenatal diagnosis by amniocentesis is even more recent. This technique can predict, in some instances, if a child will be born with congenital deformities, such as Down's syndrome (mongolism). In certain conditions, it is 98 percent accurate and considered very safe. "We can tell parents what the risks are. We deal in probabilities," one genetic counselor said. "If there is a family history of Huntington's disease, for example, we can tell the couple what the probabilities are for their child having that disease. Then they can make their own decision. A mark of a good genetic counselor is one who allows the patient to make his own decision."

In a number of disorders there is testing that can determine if one or both of the parents is actually a carrier of a specific syndrome. Tay-Sachs disease, sickle cell anemia, and thalassemia (a deadly form of anemia) can be detected in the parent, and then a determination of what the child's chances are can be made.

However, there are in excess of two thousand inherited disorders, and the vast majority cannot be detected within the parents. Such diseases as cystic fibrosis (CF), in which both parents carry a recessive gene which transmits the disorder to the child, are not detectable. However, here is an example of what genetic counseling can offer for that disease.

1. If neither prospective parent has a history of cystic fibrosis in the family, the chance of their child having the disease is 1 in 3600.

2. If one of the prospective parents has CF in his or her family, there can be a 1 in 1800 chance the child will have it, depending on the proximity of the child to the CF carrier.

3. If there is a history of CF in the families of both prospective parents, the chance of the child having it can be increased to 1 in 9, again depending on the proximity of the child to the CF carriers.

When should you avail yourself of genetic counseling? When there is a family history of a genetic disorder, counseling should be sought. Disorders such as diabetes, mental retardation, early heart disease, and physical deformities all have a genetic link. Also, any woman over the age of thirty-five having a child should seek genetic counseling. These are precautions that should be taken, but they are not guarantees. Many children born with genetic disorders have no family histories that would suggest they would be afflicted.

What must a good genetic counselor do? First, he or she must have access to good laboratory work because many of the techniques used in this area are highly sophisticated and cannot be done well except by very experienced laboratory people. Laboratory chromosomal studies, for example, are very sophisticated. Also, the good genetic counselor must be a fundamentally good medical doctor because he or she needs very good diagnostic skills. Finally, the best genetic counseling units are backed by ancillary support personnel, such as psychiatrists, social workers, and other individuals who can aid the parents in the agonizing personal decisions which often occur in this field.

Here is a list of some of the most distinguished genetic counselors in the country. They all, of course, are medical doctors who are clinical geneticists.

GENETIC COUNSELORS

Dr. Arthur D. Bloom
Department of Pediatrics
Columbia University Medical Center
630 West 168th Street
New York, New York 10032

Dr. Robin M. Bannerman
Medical Genetics Unit
Buffalo General Hospital
Buffalo, New York 14203

Dr. Robert Desnick
Department of Pediatrics
Mt. Sinai School of Medicine
New York, New York 10029

Dr. Charles J. Epstein
Department of Pediatrics
University of California
Medical Center
San Francisco, California 94143

Dr. Murray Feingold
Center for Genetic Counseling
and Birth Defect Evaluation
Tufts–New England
Medical Center
171 Harrison Avenue
Boston, Massachusetts 02111

Dr. Park Gerald
Clinical Genetics Division
Children's Hospital Medical Center
300 Longwood Avenue
Boston, Massachusetts 02115

Dr. Judith Hall
Department of Pediatrics
University of Washington
Seattle, Washington 98195

Dr. Michael M. Kabach
(Tay-Sachs disease)
California Tay-Sachs Disease
Prevention Program
Harbor General Hospital
Torrance, California 90509

Dr. Victor A. McKusick
Department of Medicine
The Johns Hopkins University
School of Medicine
Baltimore, Maryland 21205

Dr. William Mellman
Department of Human Genetics
University of Pennsylvania
Medical School
Philadelphia, Pennsylvania 19174

*Chairman, department of
human genetics.*

Dr. Henry L. Nadler
Department of Genetics
Children's Memorial Hospital
Chicago, Illinois 60614

*Pediatrician-in-chief and
chairman, department of
pediatrics, Northwestern.*

Dr. William L. Nyhan
Biochemical Genetics Laboratory
University of California
School of Medicine
La Jolla, California 92093

Dr. John Opitz
Department of Medical Genetics
University of Wisconsin
Medical School
Madison, Wisconsin 53706

Dr. Ian H. Porter
Department of Pediatrics
Birth Defects Institute
Albany Medical College
Albany, New York 12208

Dr. Vincent Riccardi
Section of Medical Genetics
Baylor College of Medicine
Houston, Texas 77025

Dr. David Rimoin
(growth disorders)
Division of Medical Genetics
Harbor–University of California at
Los Angeles Medical Center
1000 West Carson Street
Torrance, California 90509

Dr. Leon E. Rosenberg
Department of Human Genetics
Yale University Medical School
New Haven, Connecticut 06520

Dr. R. Neil Schimke
Department of Medicine
University of Kansas Medical Center
Kansas City, Kansas 66103

Dr. Roy Schmickel
Department of Pediatrics
University of Michigan
Medical Center
Ann Arbor, Michigan 48109

Dr. David W. Smith
Department of Pediatrics
Dysmorphology Unit
University of Washington
Medical School
Seattle, Washington 98195

Dr. Miriam G. Wilson
Department of Pediatrics
University of Southern California–
Los Angeles County Medical Center
1200 North State Street
Los Angeles, California 90033

Professor of pediatrics.

Reproductive Endocrinologists

(Infertility)

The specialty of reproductive endocrinology, a certified subspecialty of obstetrics and gynecology, deals mostly with the problems of infertility among women.

The birth of Louise Brown in England on July 27, 1978 (the first child conceived outside of the mother's womb), underscored the enormous strides made in recent years in fertility research. Unfortunately, the Brown case had the potentially bad effect of giving false hope to many childless couples. While the Brown case does represent a major advance (by combining male sperm and female egg from the parents outside of the womb and then quickly placing it back into the womb once the egg was fertilized), reproductive endocrinologists are quick to point out that the Louise Brown case was exceptional and cannot be duplicated routinely.

What defines infertility? If a couple attempts to have a child for a period of a year and the female does not become pregnant, physicians consider this a sign that there may be a problem with conception. In the majority of cases the problem is with the woman; however, in 30 to 40 percent of the cases, the problem is with the male. Unfortunately, there is generally less that can be done to correct the problem with the male. Urologists generally treat male infertility problems.

Problems of infertility are increasing, with some 10 to 25 percent of U.S. couples experiencing problems of conception. One reason is that many women are choosing to have their children later in life, and women generally become less fertile after the age of twenty-five. Additionally, venereal disease, such as gonorrhea, can cause a malformation of the Fallopian tubes which transport the female eggs. Gonorrhea is now very widespread in this society.

At times the corrective procedures for infertility can be relatively simple. Increasing frequency of intercourse or cutting down on alcohol consumption may be suggested. Alcohol is well known to reduce the male sperm count, as are other drugs such as nicotine. "In 50 to 60 percent of the infertility cases we see," a reproductive endocrinologist said, "we are able to assist the couple to conceive within the first year."

At times there are congenital or acquired malformations or hormonal failures. In hormonal failures, often the problem can be corrected with drug therapy. Most drug therapies do *not* increase the risk of multiple births. Only the more drastic therapy involving a drug called Pergonal and a hormone called HCG has been connected with multiple births in about 20 percent of the women who respond to this treatment. If the problem is a malformation, surgery can often open the Fallopian tube or correct another type of physical problem.

What is crucial in infertility problems is that the physician identify correctly the cause of the problem and then prescribe the best course of action to correct it. As noted, often very conservative procedures can succeed, but sometimes, when indicated, more radical approaches are called for.

When reproductive endocrinologists are not dealing with problems of infertility, they also consult on menstrual problems and problems such as hair growth on women.

REPRODUCTIVE ENDOCRINOLOGISTS

Dr. S. Jan Behrman
William Beaumont Hospital
3601 West Thirteen Mile Road
Royal Oak, Michigan 48072

In private practice.

Dr. C. D. Christian
University of Arizona
Medical Center
Tucson, Arizona 85724

Professor and chairman, department of obstetrics and gynecology.

Dr. Melvin R. Cohen
Fertility Institute
333 East Superior Street
Chicago, Illinois 60611

Director of the Fertility Institute; clinical professor of medicine, University of Chicago Medical School.

Dr. William J. Dignam
University of California at
Los Angeles Medical Center
Los Angeles, California 90024

Professor of obstetrics and gynecology.

Dr. Celso-Ramon Garcia
Hospital of the University
of Pennsylvania
3400 Spruce Street
Philadelphia, Pennsylvania 19104

William S. Shippen, Jr., professor of reproduction; director, division of human reproduction.

Dr. Charles B. Hammond
Duke Medical Center
Durham, North Carolina 27710

Associate professor of obstetrics and gynecology.

Dr. Robert Jaffe
University of California
Medical Center
San Francisco, California 94143

Professor of obstetrics and gynecology.

Dr. Howard L. Judd
University of California at
Los Angeles Medical Center
Los Angeles, California 90024

Professor of obstetrics and gynecology.

Dr. Nathan G. Kase
Yale University Medical School
New Haven, Connecticut 06510

Professor of obstetrics and gynecology.

Dr. William LeMaire
University of Miami Medical School
Biscayne Annex
Miami, Florida 33152

Professor of obstetrics and gynecology.

Dr. Brian A. Little
MacDonald House
University Hospital
2065 Adelbert Road
Cleveland, Ohio 44106

Professor of obstetrics and gynecology; director, department of reproductive biology, Case-Western Reserve Medical School.

Dr. Paul C. MacDonald
Southwestern Medical School
Dallas, Texas 75235

Professor and chairman, department of obstetrics and gynecology; chief of obstetrics and gynecology at Parkland Memorial Hospital.

Dr. Paul G. McDonough
Reproductive Endocrinology Unit
Medical College of Georgia
Augusta, Georgia 30902

Chief of R-E Unit; professor of obstetrics and gynecology.

Dr. Luigi Mastroianni, Jr.
Hospital of the University of
Pennsylvania
3400 Spruce Street
Philadelphia, Pennsylvania 19104

Professor and chairman, department of obstetrics and gynecology.

Dr. David R. Mishell, Jr.
University of Southern California–
Los Angeles County Medical Center
1200 North State Street
Los Angeles, California 90033

*Professor of obstetrics and
gynecology.*

Dr. Frederick Naftolin
Yale University Medical School
New Haven, Connecticut 06510

*Professor and chairman, department
of obstetrics and gynecology.*

Dr. Kenneth Ryan
Boston Hospital for Women
221 Longwood Avenue
Boston, Massachusetts 02115

*Professor of obstetrics and
gynecology, Harvard; chief-of-staff
at Boston Hospital for Women.*

Dr. Antonio Scommegna
Michael Reese Hospital and
Medical Center
29th Street and Ellis Avenue
Chicago, Illinois 60616

*Professor of obstetrics and
gynecology.*

Dr. Leon Speroff
University of Oregon Health
Sciences Center
Portland, Oregon 97201

*Professor and chairman, department
of gynecology.*

Dr. Sergio C. Stone
University of California
Irvine Medical School
Orange, California 92668

*Director, department of reproductive
endocrinology and infertility;
associate professor of obstetrics
and gynecology.*

Dr. George Tagatz
University of Minnesota Hospital
Minneapolis, Minnesota 55455

*Professor of obstetrics and
gynecology.*

Dr. Luther Talbert
University of North Carolina
Medical School
Chapel Hill, North Carolina 27514

*Professor of obstetrics and
gynecology.*

Dr. Raymond Vandeweile
Columbia-Presbyterian
Medical Center
622 West 168th Street
New York, New York 10032

*Professor of obstetrics and
gynecology.*

Dr. Samuel S. C. Yen
University of California
Medical School
La Jolla, California 92093

*Chairman, department of obstetrics
and gynecology.*

Maternal-Fetal Medicine

(High-Risk Pregnancy)

More and more couples are choosing to have their children born at home. While the vast majority of couples still prefer to go to the hospital, many arguments have been advanced by proponents of home birth that home birth is not only far less expensive, but it is also safer for mother and child. While the evidence is not clear that home birth is safer than hospital birth, it is indisputable that if any risk to mother or child exists, hospital birth is preferable. In cases of high-risk pregnancies, a maternal-fetal specialist (also called a perinatologist) is vital.

What is a high-risk pregnancy? There are eight readily identifiable categories which signify when the risk to mother or child or both is unusually high.

1. *Diabetes.* If a prospective mother is diabetic, the chances of serious complications during pregnancy are increased greatly.

2. *Heart problems.* Like diabetes, a history of heart problems for the mother indicates that the pregnancy may be high-risk.

3. *Previous fetal deaths.* If a mother has given birth to children before and the fetus did not survive, this again signals a high risk.

4. *Toxemia.* This is an archaic term meaning hypertension (high

blood pressure), which may have existed before the pregnancy or may have occurred because of pregnancy.

5. *Early and repeated labor.* If a prospective mother has had a history of premature labor, this too is a signal for high risk.

6. *Bleeding in pregnancy.* This may signal a miscarriage early in pregnancy. Later bleeding may signal other complications that require careful management.

7. *Anemia in pregnancy.* This can make it difficult to supply the baby with necessary oxygen without overtaxing the already heavily taxed heart.

8. *Hemolytic disease.* This disorder, of which "RH disease" is the most serious form, occurs when the mother's antibodies destroy the baby's red blood cells. This can be fatal, but many strides have been made in the treatment of this problem.

Although these high-risk factors are well known both to physicians and many prospective parents, the major problem in maternal-fetal care is that about a third to a half of the babies who require intensive care after birth are born to mothers who appeared to be low-risk. "We just don't have any way yet to identify all of those mothers who are at high risk," one prominent maternal-fetal expert noted, "but when we know what the risks are, there is no question in my mind of the benefit of closely monitoring that pregnancy."

One of the major innovations in maternal-fetal medicine is the application of ultrasound. This allows the physician to "see" the baby in utero. A newer innovation is real-time ultrasound, which allows the physician to actually see the infant in motion, to see heartbeat in fetuses as young as five to seven weeks. "We can tell immediately with these techniques the size of the baby, his position, and, of course, we can also tell immediately if he is alive," the head of one maternal-fetal unit said.

Ultrasound has been used for obstetrical imaging for some twenty years and has thus far been found to be safe, unlike x-rays, which have been linked to high leukemia rates in the children. It should be emphasized that ultrasound does not emit any x-rays.

Maternal-fetal medicine is replete with very difficult decisions and is very exacting of the physician. Says one: "You have to give the mother and the father a lot of support through the pregnancy. We deal with difficult, chancy pregnancies, and there is a lot of stress and worry. You have to give them help. Also, you have many difficult ethical decisions. If a baby is damaged, you have to ask yourself at what point you give up on that baby. You wonder sometimes if mother nature is telling you something or if you're just interfering."

There are also difficult medical problems. When should the child be taken out? How should the mother's problem be treated without doing any damage to the fetus? Which drugs can and cannot be used in acute problems suffered by the mother? The best maternal-fetal physicians are skilled in dealing with these problems.

The following are among the most outstanding maternal-fetal specialists in the country. Some do only consultive work for particular problems, but most of them offer the full range of maternal-fetal care. When appropriate, those doctors with special expertise in certain areas are noted. Special interests in this field include: toxemia; abnormal labor; gynecological infections; nutrition; and drugs during pregnancy.

MATERNAL-FETAL SPECIALISTS

Dr. Karlis Adamsons
Women and Infants Hospital
50 Mande Street
Providence, Rhode Island 02908

Chairman, department of obstetrics and gynecology.

Dr. Frederick C. Battaglia
University of Colorado
Medical School
4200 East Ninth Avenue
Denver, Colorado 80220

Professor of obstetrics; chairman, department of pediatrics; director, division of perinatal medicine. Considered by his peers to be perhaps the foremost authority on maternal-fetal problems.

Dr. M. Carlyle Crenshaw
Duke Medical Center
Durham, North Carolina 27710

Director, division of perinatal medicine.

Dr. Thomas Dillon
Roosevelt Hospital
428 West 59th Street
New York, New York 10019

Director of obstetrics and gynecology at Roosevelt; professor of obstetrics and gynecology, Columbia Medical School.

Dr. Roger K. Freeman
University of California at
Irvine Medical Center
Orange, California 92668

Professor of obstetrics and gynecology.

Dr. Emmanuel Friedman
(abnormal labor)
Beth-Israel Hospital
Boston, Massachusetts 02215

Professor of obstetrics and gynecology, Harvard.

Dr. Fritz Fuchs (abnormal labor)
New York Hospital–Cornell
Medical Center
525 East 68th Street
New York, New York 10021

Chief of gynecology and obstetrics.

Dr. Steven Gabbe
Department of Obstetrics and
Gynecology
Hospital of the University of
Pennsylvania
3400 Spruce Street
Philadelphia, Pennsylvania 19104

Dr. Guy M. Harbert, Jr. (toxemia)
University of Virginia
Medical Center
Charlottesville, Virginia 22901

*Professor of obstetrics and
gynecology.*

Dr. Charles H. Hendricks
(abnormal labor)
University of North Carolina
Medical School
Chapel Hill, North Carolina 27514

*Professor and chairman, department
of obstetrics.*

Dr. Thomas Kirschbaum
B316 Clinical Center
Michigan State University
East Lansing, Michigan 48824

*Professor and chairman, department
of obstetrics and gynecology.*

Dr. William J. Ledger
(gynecological infections)
University of Southern California
Women's Hospital
Los Angeles, California 90033

*Professor of obstetrics and
gynecology.*

Dr. Edward L. Makowski
University of Colorado
Medical School
4200 East Ninth Avenue
Denver, Colorado 80220

*Professor of obstetrics and
gynecology.*

Dr. Roy M. Pitkin (effects of
nutrition and drugs in pregnancy)
University Hospital
Iowa City, Iowa 52242

*Professor of obstetrics and
gynecology.*

Dr. Jack A. Pritchard (toxemia)
Southwestern Medical School
University of Texas
Dallas, Texas 75235

*Gillette professor of obstetrics and
gynecology.*

Dr. Edward J. Quilligan
University of Southern California
Medical School
1200 North State Street
Los Angeles, California 90033

*Professor of obstetrics and
gynecology.*

Dr. John J. Schruefer
Georgetown University Hospital
3800 Reservoir Road, NW
Washington, District of Columbia
20007

*Professor of obstetrics and
gynecology; director,
maternal-fetal medicine division.*

Dr. Richard H. Schwartz
Division of Fetal Medicine
Hospital of the University of
Pennsylvania
Philadelphia, Pennsylvania 19104

*Director, division of fetal medicine;
professor of obstetrics and
gynecology.*

Dr. A. Elmore Seeds, Jr.
University of Cincinnati
Medical Center
231 Bethesda Avenue
Cincinnati, Ohio 45267

*Professor and chairman, department
of obstetrics and gynecology.*

Dr. Frederick P. Zuspan (toxemia)
University Hospital
Columbus, Ohio 43210

*Professor and chairman, department
of obstetrics and gynecology.*

Neonatology

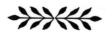

(Intensive Infant Care)

Neonatology is the specialty that deals with intensive care of babies born prematurely or with congenital defects.

This field has made enormous strides in the past few years in keeping alive children who, only a decade ago, would almost certainly have died.

About 1 percent of the births in this country every year require intensive neonatal care. At one time there were more centers than there are now because many of the centers in smaller communities have closed due to the decreased number of births. In very recent years, there has been a strong trend toward regionalization of these neonatal centers.

Although neonatal care is a crisis situation, in nearly two-thirds of the cases there is prior indication that the child may be born with problems. A mother who has had previous premature births, a diabetic mother, or a mother with high blood pressure may give birth to a child that will require intensive care at birth.

What is perhaps most astonishing in this field is how many premature babies can now be saved. Thirty years ago babies born weighing less than three pounds did not survive. Today, almost all babies born at two pounds or more survive.

With this progress have come many ethical problems. Should every possible effort be exerted to save a child who weighs only a pound even though there is less than a one in a thousand chance to save him? Should every effort be made to save a child with irreversible brain damage? New diagnostic equipment, such as the CAT scanner, now allows the diagnosis of serious brain disorders and presents this field with difficult and agonizing choices. "There is no way we can make these decisions," one noted neonatologist remarked. "I think of myself as the servant. I present the case to the family; sometimes they invite their clergyman to be with them. Once we have laid out the facts, it is up to them to make up their mind. I give them the option of choosing."

Listed are some of the most outstanding neonatologists in the country.

NEONATOLOGISTS

Dr. Billy F. Andrews
Health Sciences Center
Louisville, Kentucky 40202
Professor and chairman, department of pediatrics.

Dr. Peter Auld
New York Hospital–Cornell
Medical Center
New York, New York 10016
Director of neonatology.

Dr. Gordon B. Avery
Children's Hospital National
Medical Center
Washington, District of Columbia 20010
Director of nursery services.

Dr. Mary Ellen Avery
Children's Hospital Medical Center
Boston, Massachusetts 02115
Chief of pediatrics.

Dr. Charles Bauer
Jackson Memorial Hospital
Miami, Florida 33136
Chief of neonatology.

Dr. Richard Behrman
Rainbow Babies and Childrens
Hospital
Cleveland, Ohio 44106
Professor and chairman, department of pediatrics, Case-Western Reserve; director of pediatrics at the Rainbow Babies and Childrens Hospital.

Dr. June Brady
Children's Hospital
3700 California Street
San Francisco, California 94118
Assistant clinical professor of pediatrics, University of California; chief of neonatology at Children's Hospital.

Dr. Alfred Brann
Emory University Hospitals
Atlanta, Georgia 30303
Chief of neonatology.

Dr. George Brumley
Duke Medical Center
Durham, North Carolina 27710
Professor of pediatrics.

Dr. William Fox
Children's Hospital
Philadelphia, Pennsylvania 19104

Chief of neonatology.

Dr. Ivan D. Frantz III
Children's Hospital
Boston, Massachusetts 02115

*Physician-in-charge of newborn
ICU.*

Dr. Lawrence Gartner
Albert Einstein Medical School
Bronx, New York 10461

*Professor of pediatrics; director
of newborn services, Einstein and
and Bronx Municipal hospitals.*

Dr. Louis Gluck
University Hospital
225 West Dickinson Street
San Diego, California 92103

*Professor of pediatrics,
University of California.*

Dr. Joan E. Hodgman
Los Angeles County–University
of Southern California Medical
Center
Los Angeles, California 90033

Professor of pediatrics.

Dr. W. Alan Hodson
University of Washington
Medical School
Seattle, Washington 98195

*Director of neonatology and
professor of pediatrics, University
of Washington.*

Dr. L. Stanley James
Babies Hospital
Columbia-Presbyterian
Medical Center
New York, New York 10032

*Director, division of perinatology;
professor of pediatrics, obstetrics,
and gynecology.*

Dr. Marshall Klaus
Case-Western Reserve
Medical School
Cleveland, Ohio 44106

*Director of pediatrics, Mt. Sinai
Hospital; director of nurseries,
Case-Western Reserve.*

Dr. Jerold F. Lucey
Mary Fletcher Hospital
Burlington, Vermont 05401

*Head of neonatology; professor
of pediatrics, University of Vermont.*

Dr. Henry Nadler
Children's Memorial Hospital
Chicago, Illinois 60614

*Pediatrician-in-chief;
chairman, department of pediatrics,
Northwestern University.*

Dr. William L. Oh
Women's and Infants' Hospital
Providence, Rhode Island 02908

*Pediatrician-in-chief; professor
of pediatrics and obstetrics,
Brown University.*

Dr. Thomas K. Oliver, Jr.
Children's Hospital
Pittsburgh, Pennsylvania 15213

*Professor and chairman, department
of pediatrics, University of
Pittsburgh.*

Dr. Roderic H. Phibbs
University of California
Medical Center
San Francisco, California 94148

Director of the newborn nursery.

Dr. R. S. Pildes
Cook County Hospital
Chicago, Illinois 60612

*Chairman, department of
neonatology.*

Dr. Arnold J. Rudolph
Texas Medical Center
Houston, Texas 77025

*Professor of pediatrics, obstetrics,
and gynecology; head, newborn
section.*

Dr. Michael Simmons
Johns Hopkins Medical School
Baltimore, Maryland 21205

Dr. Mildred Stahlman
Vanderbilt Medical Center
Nashville, Tennessee 37232

*Professor of pediatrics; director,
Neonatal Lung Center.*

Dr. James M. Sutherland
Cincinnati Children's Hospital
Cincinnati, Ohio 45229

Director, newborn nursery.

Dr. H. William Taeusch, Jr.
Boston Hospital for Women
Boston, Massachusetts 02114

*Director, joint program in
neonatology.*

Dr. William Tooley
University of California
Medical Center
San Francisco, California 94143

Professor of pediatrics.

Dr. Joseph Warshaw
Yale University Medical School
New Haven, Connecticut 06510

*Chief of neonatology; professor
of pediatrics.*

PART III

Pediatric Specialists

Cardiovascular Disorders

Pediatric Cardiologists

Because of the remarkable advances in pediatric heart surgery, the most important decision to be made by pediatric cardiologists is when, and if, heart surgery should be performed on a child. One noted cardiologist said: "It is vital for the cardiologist to be an independent agent. He must not be dependent on the surgeon. He must exercise his own judgment in evaluating children for surgery. I'm afraid there are cases where some heart surgeons have had cardiologists in their pockets, and the independent judgment was often lost."

If a cardiologist does believe surgery is necessary and recommends a surgeon, it is up to the parent to ask on what basis he is recommending the surgeon. If he does not have specific answers, or does not answer you after you insist on an answer, then you may well wish to consult with another cardiologist. Any cardiologist who recommends a heart surgeon should know a number of important facts about him.

For example, he should know how many procedures of the type your child needs he has done. He should know his surgical volume—one a week is an absolute minimum. He should know his success rate in the type of procedure that is needed. He should have knowledge of the team around the surgeon because heart surgery is a total team effort. Repair of congenital defects can often be a very technically demanding procedure, much more so than a coronary by-pass, for example, and surgical expertise and experience is vital. The cardiologist must have these facts in hand.

In cases where surgery is not indicated, yet a heart problem is detected, such as a murmur or rhythm disturbance, cardiologists can often use noninvasive methods to determine the cause of the problem. They can determine if it is a "functional" disorder—that is, that while the disorder may have some symptoms, the symptoms do not indicate any defect or disease. Drug therapies are available, when indicated, for some of these problems.

Pediatric cardiologists do not subspecialize. However, two of the cardiologists listed are noted for their special interest in electrophysiology problems and rhythm disturbances.

PEDIATRIC CARDIOLOGISTS

Dr. Mary Ellen Engle
New York Hospital–Cornell
Medical Center
525 East 68th Street
New York, New York 10021

*Professor of pediatrics;
director of pediatric cardiology.*

Dr. David Fixler
Department of Pediatrics
Southwestern Medical School
Dallas, Texas 75235

Professor of pediatrics.

Dr. Henry Gelband
(rhythm abnormalities)
Department of Pediatrics
University of Miami Medical School
Miami, Florida 33152

Professor of pediatrics.

Dr. Welton M. Gersony
Columbia-Presbyterian
Medical Center
630 West 168th Street
New York, New York 10032

*Professor of pediatrics;
director, division of cardiology.*

Dr. Ira N. Gessner
University of Florida
Medical School
Gainesville, Florida 32610

*Chief, division of pediatric
cardiology; professor of pediatrics.*

Dr. Paul Gillette
(rhythm abnormalities)
Baylor College of Medicine
Houston, Texas 77030

Professor of pediatrics.

Dr. Stanley J. Goldberg
1501 North Campbell
Tucson, Arizona 85724

*Professor of pediatric cardiology,
University of Arizona.*

Dr. Warren G. Guntheroth
University of Washington
Medical School
Seattle, Washington 98195

*Head, division of pediatric
cardiology; professor of pediatrics.*

Dr. Samuel Kaplan
Children's Hospital
Cincinnati, Ohio 45229

*Professor of pediatrics;
director, division of cardiology.*

Dr. Martin H. Lees
University of Oregon Health
Sciences Center
Portland, Oregon 97201

Professor of pediatrics.

Dr. Jerome Liebman
Rainbow Babies and
Childrens Hospital
Cleveland, Ohio 44106

Professor of pediatrics.

Dr. Russell Lucas, Jr.
University of Minnesota Hospital
Minneapolis, Minnesota 55455

*Professor of pediatrics and
pediatric cardiology.*

Dr. Paul Lurie
Children's Hospital
Los Angeles, California 90027

*Head, division of cardiology;
professor of pediatrics, University
of Southern California.*

Dr. Carolyn McCue
Medical College of Virginia
Richmond, Virginia 23298

*Professor of pediatrics; director
of pediatric cardiology.*

Dr. Dan G. McNamara
Texas Children's Hospital
Houston, Texas 77030

Professor of pediatrics, Baylor.

Dr. Alexander Nadas
Children's Hospital Medical Center
Boston, Massachusetts 02115

Professor of pediatrics, Harvard.

Dr. Milton H. Paul
Children's Memorial Hospital
Chicago, Illinois 60614

Director, division of cardiology.

Dr. William Plauth, Jr.
Emory University Hospital
Atlanta, Georgia 30303

Professor of pediatrics.

Dr. William J. Rashkind
Dr. J. Sidney Freeman
Children's Hospital
Philadelphia, Pennsylvania 19104

*Dr. Rashkind is director of the
cardiovascular laboratory and
sees a limited number of patients.
Dr. Freeman does
more clinical work.*

Dr. James L. Reynolds
4440 Magnolia Street
Suite 316
New Orleans, Louisiana 70115

*Associate professor of pediatrics,
Tulane.*

Dr. Donald G. Ritter
Mayo Clinic
Rochester, Minnesota 55901

Dr. Amon Rosenthal
University of Michigan
Medical Center
Ann Arbor, Michigan 48104

Professor of pediatrics.

Dr. Abe Rudolph
University of California
Medical Center
San Francisco, California 94143

Director, department of pediatric cardiology.

Dr. Herbert D. Ruttenberg
University of Utah Medical Center
Salt Lake City, Utah 84112

Associate professor and chairman, division of cardiology.

Dr. Lewis P. Scott III
Children's Hospital–National
Medical Center
111 Michigan Avenue, NW
Washington, District of Columbia
20010

Chief of pediatric cardiology.

Dr. William Strong
Medical College of Georgia
Augusta, Georgia 30902

Dr. Norman Talner
Yale University Medical School
New Haven, Connecticut 06510

Professor of pediatrics.

Dr. Peter Vlad
Children's Hospital
Buffalo, New York 14222

Professor of pediatrics, State University of New York.

Pediatric Heart Surgeons

The major difference between pediatric heart surgeons and adult heart surgeons is that pediatric surgeons usually repair congenital defects rather than acquired heart problems. Pulmonic stenosis, septal defects, as well as more complex congenital heart defects are being repaired and in a vast number of cases insuring the child a normal life expectancy. One type of acquired heart defect pediatric heart surgeons do repair is caused by rheumatic heart disease. This usually involves repair of a heart valve. "The most significant changes in pediatric heart surgery over the past few years," one pediatric heart surgeon said, "is that we have become very aggressive and capable in repairing complex congenital heart defects in infancy."

Eight out of every 1,000 children born live in this country have congenital heart defects, and of those 8, an average of 2.5 have a "critical" disease, which means that surgery must often be performed while the child is only a few hours or at most a few days old. The advances in this area have been startling. "One of the major advantages of this type of very early surgical intervention," a heart surgeon noted, "is that we often prevent the child from dying of his heart defect, and we also prevent detrimental secondary changes to him that would have resulted if he had not had the surgery early."

There are few heart surgeons who specialize solely in pediatric heart surgery. Many of those listed here perform pediatric heart surgery only, but a few perform both adult and pediatric, and they appear on the adult list also. However, all are recognized by their peers as outstanding pediatric cardiac surgeons.

As in adult heart surgery, it is considered good medicine to have an evaluation by a cardiologist who is independent of the heart surgeon. If he or she considered surgery a necessity, and a further evaluation by the heart surgeon confirms it, that is reasonable assurance that surgery is indicated. But you may wish to seek other consultations. As in all the specialties, the surgeons listed here are chosen not only for their technical skill, but also for their surgical judgment.

PEDIATRIC HEART SURGEONS

Dr. Aldo R. Castaneda
Children's Hospital Medical Center
Boston, Massachusetts 02115

Professor of surgery, Harvard.

Dr. Gordon K. Danielson, Jr.
Mayo Clinic
Rochester, Minnesota 55901

Professor of surgery.

Dr. Paul A. Ebert
University of California
Medical Center
San Francisco, California 94143

Professor and chairman, department of surgery.

Dr. John W. Kirklin
University of Alabama
Medical Center
University Station
Birmingham, Alabama 35294

Chairman, department of surgery.

Dr. George Lindesmith
Children's Hospital
Los Angeles, California 90027

Chief, division of thoracic and cardiovascular surgery.

Dr. Dwight C. McGoon
Mayo Clinic
Rochester, Minnesota 55901

Professor of surgery, Mayo.

Dr. James R. Malm
Columbia-Presbyterian
Medical Center
161 Fort Washington Avenue
New York, New York 10032

Professor of clinical surgery.

Dr. Albert Pacifico
University of Alabama
Medical Center
University Station
Birmingham, Alabama 35294

Professor of surgery.

Dr. Albert Starr
University of Oregon
Health Science Center
Portland, Oregon 97201

*Chief, division of
cardiopulmonary surgery.*

Dr. George A. Trusler
Hospital for Sick Children
Toronto, Ontario
Canada M5G 1X8

Chief of cardiovascular surgery.

Pediatric Hypertension Specialists

The pediatric high blood pressure specialists listed here are, for the most part, nephrologists (kidney specialists) who have a special interest in high blood pressure in young children.

One reason that kidney specialists naturally have special interest in this disorder is because kidney disease, such as chronic kidney infections or disease of a kidney artery, can also cause high blood pressure. In young people, abnormal growth of a portion of a kidney artery wall may be the cause of the high blood pressure, a congenital condition which can be repaired by surgery, performed usually by vascular surgeons or pediatric urologists.

There is also little doubt that high blood pressure, at least in part, is an inherited disorder, and in some cases children at an early age can have substantial high blood pressure because of genetic factors. Drug and diet therapies are available to control hypertension in cases where blood pressures are high enough to require treatment.

Hypertension has been detected in very young children, some as young as three or four, but specialists warn that one reading of an elevated pressure does not necessarily mean the child is hypertensive. However, they do say that the child should be followed closely to see if his or her readings continue to be high. If they do, the child must be considered hypertensive.

What constitutes a high reading for blood pressure in children? There is no broad agreement as to when a child should be labeled hypertensive. Blood pressures that are "high normal" for his or her age should be watched over a period of time to see if they remain high. Readings of 130/85 or 135/85 are in a "gray" area because while they are high, they do not mean unequivocally that the child is hypertensive. However, continued readings of 140/90 (a borderline reading for adults) should be interpreted to mean that the child is suffering from high blood pressure and should be evaluated by a specialist.

The top number (140) is the systolic pressure, the pressure on the artery walls when the heart beats. The bottom number (90) is the diastolic pressure (when the heart is at rest between beats).

Although high blood pressure is usually symptomless, it is a serious medical condition that, if left ignored, can have grave consequences. In a study in Evans County, Georgia, 11 percent of 435 teen-agers examined were found to have high blood pressure. Only seven years later, the investigators tracked down thirty of those teen-agers with hypertension who had *not* been treated. They found two had already died of strokes, one had heart disease, three had developed brain and heart symptoms, and five others had no symptoms as yet, but their pressures were more elevated.

PEDIATRIC HYPERTENSION SPECIALISTS

Dr. David Goldring
Children's Hospital
St. Louis, Missouri 63178

Professor of pediatrics;
Washington University
Medical School.

Dr. Ira Greifer
Albert Einstein Medical School
Bronx, New York 10461

Associate professor of pediatrics.

Dr. Alan B. Gruskin
St. Christopher's Hospital
Philadelphia, Pennsylvania 19133

Professor of pediatrics, Temple
University Medical School.

Dr. Malcolm A. Holliday
Children's Renal Center
400 Parnassus Avenue
San Francisco, California 94143

Professor of pediatrics, University
of California Medical School.

Dr. Julie R. Ingelfinger
Children's Hospital Medical Center
Boston, Massachusetts 02115

Assistant professor of
pediatrics, Harvard.

Dr. Ellin Lieberman
Children's Hospital
Los Angeles, California 90054

Associate professor; head,
division of pediatric nephrology,
University of Southern California.

Dr. Jennifer M. H. Loggie
Children's Hospital
Research Foundation
Cincinnati, Ohio 45229

Professor of pediatrics, University
of Cincinnati Medical School.

Dr. Bernard Mirkin
University of Minnesota Hospitals
Minneapolis, Minnesota 55455

Professor of pediatrics and
pharmacology.

Dr. Maria I. New
525 East 68th Street
New York, New York 10021

*Chairwoman, department of
pediatrics, Cornell Medical School.*

Dr. Alan Sinaiko
University of Minnesota Hospitals
Minneapolis, Minnesota 55455

*Associate professor of pediatrics
and pharmacology.*

Pulmonary Specialists

Asthma, Cystic Fibrosis, and Other Lung Disorders

A number of pulmonary disorders can strike children, but perhaps the most common serious complaint seen by pediatric pulmonary specialists results from complicated asthma cases.

Asthma, which is also treated by allergists, can in some cases be fatal because of the effects this disease has on the breathing passages.

Another serious disorder which pulmonary specialists often treat is cystic fibrosis, or CF. CF is an inherited systemic disease. Today, many CF victims are now enjoying longer and better lives because of treatment. At one time, CF victims almost always died by their teens; now there are many who live into their twenties, thirties, and even forties.

Because it attacks many systems of the body, many different types of specialists have an interest in CF, including gastroenterologists and allergists. Although the complications from the disease are numerous, the evidence is convincing that children treated for CF at medical centers or by experts in this field have significantly longer life spans and significantly fewer complications. "There is no question," one CF expert said, "that the children who get the proper treatment and whose parents are educated properly in the care of their child do much, much better than children who do not have the benefit of this care."

CF centers are now located at most children's hospitals and at most major medical centers and larger hospitals.

Pulmonary specialists also treat TB, complications from congenital lung deformities, lung infections, and a number of other disorders.

Some of the specialists listed here head CF units in their medical centers and they treat CF patients as a major part of their clinical care. Others offer more general pediatric pulmonary care. In a few cases, the specialist listed is not in pulmonary medicine, but is listed here because he or she directs a cystic fibrosis center.

PEDIATRIC PULMONARY SPECIALISTS

Dr. Mary Ellen Avery
Children's Hospital Medical Center
Boston, Massachusetts 02115

Professor of pediatrics, Harvard; especially known for her expertise in newborn lung disease.

Dr. Giulio Barbero
University of Missouri
Medical Center
Columbia, Missouri 65210

Professor and chairman, department of pediatrics. Dr. Barbero is a gastroenterologist, not a pulmonary specialist, but is listed here because he heads the cystic fibrosis clinic.

Dr. Harvey Colten
Children's Hospital Medical Center
Boston, Massachusetts 02115

Professor of pediatrics and chief of the cystic fibrosis clinic. Dr. Colten is an allergist, not a pulmonary specialist, but is listed here because he heads the CF clinic.

Dr. Ernest K. Cotton
University of Colorado
Medical Center
Denver, Colorado 80220

Director, division of pediatric pulmonary medicine.

Dr. Murray Davidson
Long Island Jewish
Hillside Medical Center
New Hyde Park, New York 11040

Dr. Davidson is a pediatric gastroenterologist but is listed here because of his expertise in cystic fibrosis.

Dr. Carolyn Denning
St. Vincent's Hospital
153 West 11th Street
New York, New York 10011

Chief of the cystic fibrosis clinic.

Dr. Paul A. DiSant'Agnese
Building 10
Room 8N250
National Institutes of Health
Bethesda, Maryland 20014

Director of the cystic fibrosis clinic. As in all National Institutes of Health care, you must be referred by a physician and your disorder must conform to the National Institutes of Health research protocols. Care is free.

Dr. Carl Doershuk
Rainbow Babies and
Childrens Hospital
Cleveland, Ohio 44106

Head of the CF center; professor of pediatrics, Case-Western Reserve.

Dr. Samuel T. Giammona
Children's Hospital
San Francisco, California 94118

Director of the pulmonary center; professor of pediatrics, University of California.

Dr. Gunyon M. Harrison
Texas Children's Hospital
Houston, Texas 77030

Director of the cystic fibrosis clinic.

Dr. Edwin Kendig
Medical College of Virginia
Richmond, Virginia 23298

Professor of pediatrics. An authority on tuberculosis.

Dr. John Mangos
University of Florida Medical Center
Gainesville, Florida 32601

Professor of pediatrics. Noted primarily for his research into cystic fibrosis, but sees some patients on a consulting basis.

Dr. Leroy Matthews
Rainbow Babies and
Childrens Hospital
Cleveland, Ohio 44106

Professor of pediatrics, Case Western Reserve. An authority on CF. Sees some patients on a consulting basis.

Dr. Robert Mellins
Columbia-Presbyterian
Medical Center
New York, New York 10032

Professor of pediatrics.

Dr. Robert H. Schwartz
Strong Memorial Hospital
Rochester, New York 14642

Director of the cystic fibrosis center.

Dr. Daniel Shannon
Massachusetts General Hospital
Boston, Massachusetts 02114

Associate professor of pediatrics. A special interest in sudden infant death syndrome.

Dr. Harry Shwachman
Children's Hospital Medical Center
Boston, Massachusetts 02115

Professor of pediatrics, Harvard. One of the major figures in cystic fibrosis. Sees patients only on a consulting basis.

Dr. Alexander Spock
Duke University Medical Center
Durham, North Carolina 27710

Director of the cystic fibrosis center.

Dr. Donald B. Strominger
Children's Hospital
St. Louis, Missouri 63178

Director of the cystic fibrosis center.

Dr. Richard Talamo
The Johns Hopkins Hospital
Baltimore, Maryland 21205

Heads the CF center; professor of pediatrics.

Dr. Lynn M. Taussig
University of Arizona
Medical Center
Tucson, Arizona 85274

Director of pediatric pulmonary disease section.

Dr. William Tooley
University of California
Medical Center
San Francisco, California 94143

Professor of pediatrics.

Dr. Chun-I Wang
Cystic Fibrosis Center
Children's Hospital
Los Angeles, California 90054

Center director.

Dr. William W. Warring
Tulane University Medical School
New Orleans, Louisiana 70112

*Chief of pediatric pulmonary
disease section.*

Disorders of the
Nervous System

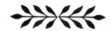

Neurological Disorders

Pediatric neurologists treat a wide range of childhood neurologic disorders, including hyperactivity, epilepsy, dyslexia, as well as a number of other rarer disorders.

Few pediatric neurologists confine their work to special areas, but many have special interests in certain disorders. These are:

Epilepsy disorders. This is the most common condition that pediatric neurologists encounter, and everyone listed here has had wide experience in diagnosing and treating it. Epilepsy causes intermittent disturbances of consciousness and other neurological functions. In all except the most extreme cases, it can be managed with appropriate drug therapy.

Muscle diseases. Muscular dystrophies and muscle inflammation are two of the neurological disorders which would come under this special area of interest.

Reye's syndrome. A condition that follows a viral infection, it causes acute swelling of the brain. Untreated, only 20 percent of the children who contract it survive. If diagnosed early and treated aggressively, 70 to 80 percent survive.

Headache. Complex headache problems, such as migraine in childhood, can require specialized care.

Communication disorders. Difficulties of speech or understanding fall under this category.

Degenerative or metabolic neurologic diseases. Such diseases as Tay-Sachs would be included. Usually there is little that can be done to reverse the process of the disease, but accurate identification of the specific disease is important for genetic counseling of the parents should they decide to have another child.

Other special interests include brain tumors, hydrocephalus (commonly called water on the brain), as well as infectious diseases of the nervous system.

PEDIATRIC NEUROLOGISTS

Dr. Charles F. Barlow (epilepsy)
Children's Hospital Medical Center
Boston, Massachusetts 02115

Bronson Crothers professor of neurology, Harvard.

Dr. William E. Bell (brain tumors)
Department of Pediatrics
and Neurology
University of Iowa Hospitals
Iowa City, Iowa 52242

Professor of pediatrics and neurology. His special interests also include neurologic infections, such as encephalitis and meningitis, which affect the nervous system.

Dr. Bruce Berg
University of California
Medical Center
San Francisco, California 94143

Associate professor of pediatrics and neurology.

Dr. Peter Berman
Children's Hospital
Philadelphia, Pennsylvania 19104

Associate professor of neurology and pediatrics, University of Pennsylvania.

Dr. Abe M. Chutorian
Neurological Institute
710 West 168th Street
New York, New York 10032

Dr. Darryl DeVivo
(Reye's syndrome)
Neurological Institute
710 West 168th Street
New York, New York 10032

Dr. DeVivo is head of pediatric neurology.

Dr. Philip R. Dodge
St. Louis Children's Hospital
St. Louis, Missouri 63110

Professor and chairman, department of pediatrics, Washington University.

Dr. Margaret Caroline Duncan
Louisiana State University
Medical School
1542 Tulane Avenue
New Orleans, Louisiana 70112

Professor of pediatrics and neurology.

Dr. Paul R. Dyken
(neuromuscular diseases)
Medical College of Georgia
Augusta, Georgia 30902

*Professor of neurology and
pediatrics. Also has a special
interest in epilepsy.*

Dr. Gerald M. Fenichel
(muscle diseases)
Vanderbilt Medical Center
Nashville, Tennessee 37232

*Professor and chairman,
department of neurology.*

Dr. John Freeman (epilepsy)
The Johns Hopkins Hospital
Baltimore, Maryland 21205

*Professor of pediatrics and
neurology. Also noted for his
expertise in congenital
neurologic defects in infants,
such as hydrocephalus.*

Dr. Joseph H. French
(degenerative neurologic diseases)
Montefiore Hospital
Bronx, New York 10467

*Professor of neurology and
pediatrics.*

Dr. Manuel R. Gomez
Mayo Clinic
Rochester, Minnesota 55901

Professor of pediatric neurology.

Dr. Leonard Graziani
Jefferson Medical College
Philadelphia, Pennsylvania 19102

*Professor of pediatrics and
neurology.*

Dr. Robert V. Groover
Mayo Clinic
Rochester, Minnesota 55901

Dr. Ray W. Mackey
University of Texas Medical School
San Antonio, Texas 78284

*Professor of pediatrics and
neurology.*

Dr. John H. Menkes
(degenerative brain diseases)
9615 Brighton Way
Beverly Hills, California 90210

*Clinical professor of pediatrics
and neurology, University of
Southern California.*

Dr. Isabelle Rapin
(communication disorders)
Albert Einstein College of Medicine
Bronx, New York 10461

*Professor of neurology and
pediatrics. Also known for her
interest in hyperactivity and
degenerative brain diseases.*

Dr. N. Paul Rosman
(headache disorders)
Boston City Hospital
Boston, Massachusetts 02118

*Professor of pediatrics and
neurology, Boston University.
Also noted for his interest in
head injuries.*

Dr. James F. Schwartz (infections)
Emory University Medical School
Atlanta, Georgia 30303

*Professor of pediatrics and
neurology. Also has a special
interest in acute encephalitis.*

Dr. Alfred J. Spiro
(muscle diseases)
Albert Einstein College of Medicine
Bronx, New York 10461

*Associate professor of neurology
and pediatrics.*

Dr. Kenneth F. Swaiman
(muscle diseases)
University of Minnesota
Medical School
Minneapolis, Minnesota 55455

*Professor and director, division of
pediatric neurology.*

Dr. John J. Volpe
(newborn neurologic disorders)
St. Louis Children's Hospital
St. Louis, Missouri 63110

*Associate professor of pediatrics
and neurology. Known for his
expertise in diagnosis, prognosis,
and treatment of newborn and
prematurely born infants with
neurological disorders.*

Dr. Gordon Watters
McGill University Medical School
Montreal, Quebec
Canada

*Associate professor of neurology
and pediatrics.*

Pediatric Neurosurgeons

Hydrocephalus (water on the brain) was at one time an untreatable condition. Today there have been remarkable advances made in surgical correction of this congenital disorder. This condition is one of the areas in which pediatric neurosurgeons concentrate. Also, such congenital conditions as abnormal cranial or spinal development, congenital tumors, brain tumors, and a condition called meningomyelocele, a condition which causes water sacs on the back, can to a significant extent be corrected.

The neurosurgeons listed here perform pediatric neurosurgery exclusively. The most obvious major difference between adult neurosurgery and pediatric neurosurgery is the concentration on repair of congenital defects in pediatric work. The surgeons listed here perform the full range of pediatric neurosurgery.

PEDIATRIC NEUROSURGEONS

Dr. E. Bruce Hendrick
Hospital for Sick Children
Toronto, Ontario
Canada M5G 1X8

Dr. Mark S. O'Brien
Emory University Clinic
Atlanta, Georgia 30322

*Professor of surgery
(neurosurgery).*

Dr. Anthony Raimondi
Children's Memorial Hospital
Chicago, Illinois 60614

Professor of neurosurgery,
Northwestern University.

Dr. Luis Schut
Children's Hospital
Philadelphia, Pennsylvania 19104

Associate professor of
neurosurgery.

Dr. M. Peter Sayers
Children's Hospital
Columbus, Ohio 43205

Clinical professor of surgery
(neurosurgery), Ohio State.

Dr. John Shillito, Jr.
Children's Hospital Medical Center
Boston, Massachusetts 02115

Associate professor of
surgery, Harvard.

Child Psychiatrists

When does a child need the attention of a child psychiatrist? There are no absolute answers to this question, but in general child psychiatrists suggest that parents should be especially aware when certain behaviors become persistent and severe.

Childhood depression, only very recently recognized as a diagnosable disorder, is perhaps the newest psychiatric problem known to affect children. "The myth of childhood being a necessarily happy, carefree period of life has prejudiced even some psychiatrists," remarked one child psychiatrist, and he adds that there are many instances of depression in very young children.

What may be signs of clinical childhood depression and other childhood disorders?

1. If the child is unable to have fun, refuses to eat his or her favorite food, and is otherwise miserable for a month or more without an obvious explanation, such as a death in the family, then this may be a signal that he or she needs experienced professional help. Other signs may include complaints of being tired all the time yet not sleeping, continued talk about dying, and frequent crying.

2. The child is unable to have experiences that are right for that stage of life. For example, he or she is too shy to go to school or has phobias that would be normal for a two-year-old but not normal for for a ten-year-old.

3. He or she has no friends or always fights with the friends he has.

4. He or she fights with his siblings and the fighting causes serious injury.

5. Difficulty in school that causes the child to be two grade levels behind his peers can be a sign of a serious learning disorder.

"It's often a question of good judgment," one prominent child psychiatrist said, "but it should be kept in mind that some types of behaviors that are abnormal for children in one family would not be abnormal for children in another family. It is important to know and understand the child's background before deciding whether or not his behavior is inappropriate. Also, what might be inappropriate behavior for a child of ten may be perfectly appropriate behavior for a child of four. So the age of the child is also very important."

There are a number of other mental and emotional disorders that strike children and that are more obviously in need of treatment: serious communication or perceptual disorders, antisocial behavior, sexual identification problems, anorexia nervosa (not eating), autism, and a number of other problems peculiar to childhood. The leading child psychiatrists listed here have special interest in many of these problems.

However, it is well to keep in mind that all of them are generalists. They all treat the full range of childhood problems usually in all age ranges, from infancy to adolescence. However, some are known for their interest in problems of infancy, and others in adolescent problems. Perhaps the single most common emotional problem confronted by child psychiatrists (and child neurologists) is hyperactivity. Those noted in this special field caution that hyperactivity is in fact a "very rare" disorder which has come into vogue only recently and therefore has led to widespread misdiagnosis. Many children who are labeled hyperactive, and given drugs for it, are not in fact hyperactive, they contend. "The actual disorder of hyperactivity is not common," one child psychiatrist noted, "but it gets used a lot because teachers and school administrators don't know what else to call kids who won't pay attention in class. So many kids get stuck with the label when the problem is really something else."

Perhaps the single most important aspect of child psychiatry as opposed to adult psychiatry is to realize that children are "in process," that is, they are still forming and going through stages, and that certain behaviors can and will improve with time. Also, child psychiatrists seek to relate to children in nonmedical settings, and they should seek to establish bridges to the parents, teachers, and others who may be directly involved in the child's life. "A good child psychiatrist must be able to deal well with adults," a child psychiatrist noted, "because ultimately the child is in the care of adults."

In some cases outpatient psychiatric care is not sufficient and residential treatment (inpatient care) is required. Although the criteria for determining when a child should be institutionalized are made on a case-by-case basis, there are some basic guidelines for nonemergency residential care.

1. If the child is failing significantly in three major areas—home, school, and neighborhood—then he or she may benefit from residential treatment.

2. If there has been an honest effort at correcting the child's problem on an outpatient basis but it has failed, then residential treatment may be considered.

3. If there is a facility which has a special competence for the individual child's problem, then this may offer him the best opportunity for recovery.

Child psychiatrists admit that residential treatment facilities for children are not standardized and that they vary, in the words of one psychiatrist, "from excellence to exploitation." If the credentials of the center director are excellent and the center is a member of the American Association for Children's Residential Centers, this is a positive sign. But the best method of selecting an appropriate residential treatment center is on the advice of a trusted and expert child psychiatrist.

Although all of the psychiatrists listed here are noted for their expertise in childhood disturbances and for their patient care, the interaction between the doctor and you and your child is vital.

What are signs that the "chemistry" may not be right? The most obvious is that the problem does not get any better or that you as a parent remain confused or uninformed over how the psychiatrist has diagnosed and is treating your child.

As noted, but it should be emphasized again, the eminent child psychiatrists singled out here practice general child psychiatry. Some emphasize one approach more than another, but all of them have dealt with the full range of childhood mental and emotional disorders, a range which is enormous. However, those known for a special research or clinical interest are so noted. It should also be noted that many of them are in academic institutions and do not have a heavy patient load. They do refer patients, however, as well as see a limited number of patients.

CHILD PSYCHIATRISTS

Dr. Thomas Anders
(sleep disorders; nightmares)
Children's Hospital
Stanford University Medical Center
Stanford, California 94305

Professor of child psychiatry.

Dr. E. James Anthony (children of
psychotic parents; depression)
William Greenleaf Elliott
Division of Child Psychiatry
369 North Taylor Street
St. Louis, Missouri 63108

*Director of the division; professor
of psychiatry at Washington
University Medical School.*

Dr. Meyer Bahlburg (early
effeminacy in boys; transsexualism)
Columbia-Presbyterian
Medical Center
622 West 168th Street
New York, New York 10032

Professor of psychiatry.

Dr. Norman Bernstein (mental
retardation; burns in childhood)
Department of Psychiatry
University of Illinois
912 South Wood Street
Chicago, Illinois 60612

Professor of psychiatry.

Dr. Dennis Cantwell (depression;
autism; anorexia nervosa)
Neuropsychiatric Institute
University of California at Los
Angeles Medical Center
Los Angeles, California 90024

Dr. Stella Chess
(severe perceptual handicaps)
333 East 49th Street
New York, New York 10017

*Professor of psychiatry, New York
University. Dr. Chess is noted for
her expertise in congenital
perceptual defects caused by
rubella (German measles). Dr.
Chess is retired from headship of the
child psychiatry section but
continues to see patients. She is
also known for her research into
children's temperament.*

Dr. Donald Cohen
(autistic and psychotic children)
Yale Child Study Center
Yale University Medical School
New Haven, Connecticut 06510

Dr. Richard Cohen
(juvenile delinquency)
Child Guidance Clinic
University of Pittsburgh
Pittsburgh, Pennsylvania 15213

Director of the clinic.

Dr. James Comer (effects of
prejudice on children)
Yale Child Study Center
Yale University Medical School
New Haven, Connecticut 06510

Professor of psychiatry.

Dr. James Eagan (depression;
learning disabilities)
Children's Hospital–National
Medical Center
111 Michigan Avenue, NW
Washington, District of Columbia
20010

Dr. Leon Eisenberg (drugs
and hyperactivity; autism)
Children's Hospital Medical Center
300 Longwood Avenue
Boston, Massachusetts 02115

*Professor of psychiatry, Harvard.
Dr. Eisenberg is considered an
authority on the use and misuse
of drugs in hyperactivity.*

Dr. John Fowler (hyperactivity)
Duke University Medical Center
Durham, North Carolina 27710

*Professor and chairman, division
of child psychiatry.*

Dr. Frederick Gottlieb
(family therapy)
Neuropsychiatric Institute
University of California at Los
Angeles Medical Center
Los Angeles, California 90024

Dr. Lawrence Greenberg
(hyperactivity)
University of Minnesota
Medical School
Minneapolis, Minnesota 55455

Professor of psychiatry.

Dr. Douglas Hansen (children of
divorce; school problems)
Baylor College of Medicine
Houston, Texas 77025

Director, child study clinic.

Dr. Dorothy Lewis
(juvenile delinquency)
New York Psychiatric Institute
722 West 168th Street
New York, New York 10032

Dr. Melvin Lewis
Yale Child Study Center
Yale University Medical School
New Haven, Connecticut 06510

*Professor of clinical pediatrics
and child psychiatry.*

Dr. Reginald Lourie (infancy)
The Psychiatric Institute
4460 MacArthur Boulevard, NW
Washington, District of Columbia
20007

*Dr. Lourie sees patients only on
a consulting basis.*

Dr. Jack Martin
(residential treatment)
3636 Dickason
Suite 6
Dallas, Texas 75219

Dr. Ake Mattsson (problems of
puberty; hemophiliac children)
New York University
Medical Center
550 First Avenue
New York, New York 10016

Professor of psychiatry.

Dr. Peter Neubauer (infancy)
33 East 70th Street
New York, New York 10021

*Director of the Child Development
Center at 120 West 57th Street in
New York City.*

Dr. Joseph Noshpitz (children in
residential treatment; adolescence)
Children's Hospital–National
Medical Center
111 Michigan Avenue, NW
Washington, District of Columbia
20010

*Clinical professor of psychiatry,
child health, and human
development, George Washington
University Medical School.*

Dr. Silvio Onesti
(children in residential treatment)
McClean Hospital
Belmont, Massachusetts 02178

Director of child psychiatry.

Dr. Irving Phillips (depression)
University of California
Medical Center
Third and Parnassus
San Francisco, California 94122

Professor of psychiatry.

Dr. Elva Poznanski (medically
hospitalized children; depression)
University of Michigan
Medical Center
Children's Psychiatric Hospital
Ann Arbor, Michigan 48103

Professor of psychiatry.

Dr. Dane Prugh (child abuse)
Department of Pediatrics
University of Colorado
Medical Center
4200 East Ninth Avenue
Denver, Colorado 80220

Professor of psychiatry.

Dr. Joaquim Puig-Antich
(depression)
Columbia-Presbyterian
Medical Center
622 West 168th Street
New York, New York 10023

Dr. Frank Rafferty
(antisocial children)
Institute for Juvenile Research
907 South Wolcott Avenue
Chicago, Illinois 60612

Director of the institute.

Dr. Judith Rappaport
(obsessional neuroses; hyperactivity)
Unit on Childhood Mental Illness
National Institutes of Mental Health
Clinical Center
Bethesda, Maryland 20014

*As in all National Institutes of
Health and National Institutes of
Mental Health care, there is no fee.
However, patients require referrals
from other physicians and must fit
into the established National
Institutes of Health research
protocols. For information
regarding the protocols and
whether or not you might be
eligible for treatment at the
Childhood Mental Illness Unit,
call Dr. Walter Seery,
(301) 496-5111.*

Dr. Robert Reichler
(infantile autism)
Department of Psychiatry and
Behavioral Science
University of Washington
Medical School
Seattle, Washington 98105

Professor of psychiatry.

Dr. Edward Ritvo
(autism; developmental disorders)
Neuropsychiatric Institute
University of California at Los
Angeles Medical Center
Los Angeles, California 90024

*Associate professor of child
psychiatry and mental retardation.*

Dr. Herbert Schiele
(residential treatment)
6701 Springbank Street
Philadelphia, Pennsylvania 19119

Dr. David Shaffer (epilepsy;
brain damage; bedwetting)
New York State Psychiatric Institute
722 West 168th Street
New York, New York 10032

Professor of psychiatry, Columbia.

Dr. Theodore Shapiro
(delays in speaking)
Payne Whitney Clinic
50 East 72nd Street
New York, New York 10021

Director of the clinic.

Dr. Albert Solnit (children in
adoption; childhood crises)
Yale Child Study Center
Yale University Medical School
New Haven, Connecticut 06510

*Director, child study center;
professor of psychiatry and
pediatrics.*

Dr. George Tarjan
(mental retardation)
Neuropsychiatric Institute
University of California at Los
Angeles Medical Center
Los Angeles, California 90024

Professor of psychiatry.

Dr. Stanley Walzer
Children's Hospital Medical Center
300 Longwood Avenue
Boston, Massachusetts 02115

Dr. Richard Ward
Emory University
1711 Aidmore Drive, NE
Atlanta, Georgia 30707

Professor of psychiatry.

Disorders of the
Digestive System

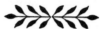

Functional and Organic Aspects of Gastrointestinal Disorders

Abdominal pain is the most frequent complaint children bring to pediatric GI specialists. Locating the source of that pain is one of the more difficult challenges in this specialty, particularly when there are no obvious causes. "The largest part of pediatric gastroenterology," one noted pediatric gastroenterologist remarked, "is to determine if the cause of the pain is from organic disease or whether it is a functional problem. The skill of the gastroenterologist is measured not just by his knowledge of organic disease, but by how well he handles the functional problems."

What is a functional problem? It is a problem that causes symptoms, such as pain, but cannot be diagnosed. Its cause may be nerves, tension, home environment, school environment, or any one of many different problems.

Another pediatric GI specialist remarked: "All illnesses have emotional aspects. It's wrong, I think, when we can't find a cause of a complaint, to say to the child or the parent that 'it's in the child's head.' The head is part of the body. The pain he feels may be a way of his coping or adjusting to life. But the pain is real and so is the problem. A variety of environmental factors may be impinging on the biological state of this individual."

A variety of organic problems can also beset children. Diarrhea, vomiting in infancy, and chronic pain are some of the more common ones.

Of a generally more serious nature are inflammatory bowel disease, colitis, ulcers, congenital GI deformities, as well as a number of liver disorders. Unlike adult GI specialists, pediatric GI specialists do not subspecialize in liver disorders, largely because of the low number of pediatric liver problems. Liver disorders, such as hepatitis and a major congenital abnormality, biliary atresia, are treated by pediatric GI specialists. Biliary atresia can now be treated surgically, but the success rate remains low. (See pediatric general surgery section.) Reye's syndrome, a liver disease which has severe neurological consequences, is also treated by pediatric GI specialists (and pediatric neurologists), as are glycogen storage disease and other genetic diseases. Cancers of the digestive system are also treated medically by pediatric GI specialists, although cancers of this region in children are relatively rare.

PEDIATRIC GASTROINTESTINAL SPECIALISTS

Dr. Marvin E. Ament
University of California at Los
Angeles Medical Center
Los Angeles, California 90024

*Associate professor of pediatrics
and medicine; chief of division of
pediatric gastroenterology.*

Dr. Giulio Barbero
University of Missouri
Medical Center
Columbia, Missouri 65210

*Professor and chairman, department
of pediatrics.*

Dr. Daniel Caplan
Emory University Hospitals
Atlanta, Georgia 30308

Chief of pediatric GI division.

Dr. Michael I. Cohen
Montefiore Hospital
Bronx, New York 10461

*Professor of pediatrics, Albert
Einstein College of Medicine;
head of pediatric GI.*

Dr. Murray Davidson
Long Island Jewish Hillside
Medical Center
New Hyde Park, New York 11040

Director of pediatric GI.

Dr. Joyce Gryboski
Yale University Medical School
New Haven, Connecticut 06510

Director of pediatric GI.

Dr. J. R. Hamilton
Hospital for Sick Children
Toronto, Ontario
Canada M5G 1X8

Head of pediatric GI.

Dr. John J. Herbst
University of Utah Medical Center
Salt Lake City, Utah 84111

*Associate professor of pediatrics;
head of pediatric GI.*

Dr. Abraham Jellin
Brookdale Hospital
Brooklyn, New York 11212

Head of pediatric GI.

Dr. William M. Michener
Cleveland Clinic
Cleveland, Ohio 44106

Head of GI services.

Dr. Claude Morin
Hospital Sainte-Justine
Montreal, Quebec
Canada H3T 1C5

Dr. John C. Partin
Children's Hospital
Cincinnati, Ohio 45229

*Professor of pediatrics, University of
Cincinnati; head of pediatric GI.*

Dr. Claude C. Roy
Hospital Sainte-Justine
Montreal, Quebec
Canada H3T 1C5

*Chief of pediatric GI; professor
of pediatrics, University of
Montreal.*

Dr. Arnold Silverman
University of Colorado
Medical Center
Denver, Colorado 80220

*Clinical professor of pediatrics;
director of pediatrics, Denver
General Hospital.*

Dr. Philip Sunshine
Stanford University Medical Center
Stanford, California 94305

*Professor of pediatrics; head of
pediatric GI.*

Dr. Michael Thaler
University of California
Medical Center
San Francisco, California 94143

Director of pediatric GI.

Dr. W. Allan Walker
Massachusetts General Hospital
Boston, Massachusetts 02114

*Chief of pediatric GI
and nutrition division.*

Dr. John Watkins
Children's Hospital
Philadelphia, Pennsylvania 19104

Head of GI services.

Diseases of the
Bones and Joints

Juvenile Arthritis

Childhood rheumatoid arthritis is quite different from adult arthritis
and must be treated differently, according to pediatric rheumatologists.
For example, although cortisone is taken by some adults to reduce the
inflammation of arthritis, this is a very risky drug for young people
to take because it stunts their growth. A direct cortisone injection into
a joint is not especially hazardous, experts say, but taking cortisone
orally can pose hazards to young people's health that may be as serious
as the disease itself. Cortisone for adults also poses some hazards. It
should also be pointed out that juvenile rheumatoid arthritis is *not*
the same as rheumatic fever, a disease with which it is often confused.

Most juvenile rheumatologists agree that the best approach to treatment of rheumatoid arthritis is a conservative one, including the
application of heat, the proper exercises, and the use of aspirin for
pain and inflammation. The progress of the child and the disorder
must be monitored carefully because in some cases the disease can
become very seriously crippling and, at times, life-threatening.

More encouraging is the fact that at least half of the children
afflicted with juvenile rheumatoid arthritis outgrow the disease. "The
major task for treatment of juvenile arthritis," one expert noted, "is
to successfully manage the disease and at the same time keep the child's
home and school life as normal as possible."

Below are listed some of the outstanding pediatric rheumatologists in the country:

PEDIATRIC RHEUMATOLOGISTS

Dr. Balu Athryea
Children's Hospital
34th Street and Civic
Center Boulevard
Philadelphia, Pennsylvania 19104

Chief of rheumatology.

Dr. John Baum
Monroe Community Hospital
435 East Henrietta Road
Rochester, New York 14603

*Professor of medicine and
pediatrics and of preventive
medicine and community health,
University of Rochester
Medical School.*

Dr. Earl Brewer, Jr.
Texas Children's Hospital
6621 Fannin Street
Houston, Texas 77030

Director, rheumatology clinic.

Dr. John J. Calabro
Saint Vincent's Hospital
25 Winthrop Street
Worcester, Massachusetts 01604

*Professor of medicine and pediatrics
at the University of Massachusetts.*

Dr. Chester W. Fink
Southwestern Medical School
5323 Harry Hines Boulevard
Dallas, Texas 75235

Professor of internal medicine.

Dr. V. Hanson
Children's Hospital
4650 Sunset Boulevard
Los Angeles, California 90027

*Professor of pediatrics, University
of Southern California.*

Dr. Jerry C. Jacobs
Babies Hospital
Columbia University Medical Center
166th Street and Broadway
New York, New York 10032

*Associate clinical professor of
pediatrics.*

Dr. Joseph E. Levinson
Division of Rheumatology
Cincinnati General Hospital
Cincinnati, Ohio 45267

*Professor of medicine, associate
professor of pediatrics, University
of Cincinnati College of Medicine.*

Dr. Jane Green Schaller
University of Washington
School of Medicine
Seattle, Washington 98195

Professor of pediatrics.

Pediatric Orthopedic Surgeons

The conditions most frequently treated by pediatric orthopedic surgeons include surgery for juvenile rheumatoid arthritis, spinal cord injuries, and scoliosis (spine curvature). In addition, pediatric orthopedic surgeons perform surgical procedures on children with cerebral palsy. Many of these procedures have made substantial strides in the past few years in both alleviating these conditions and curing them.

Congenital abnormalities of the hands and feet are also repaired. One of the most frequent foot conditions is clubfoot. Also, some children are born with hip abnormalities, such as a hip out of the socket or a condition called Perethes disease, where the hip is damaged. This occurs in children at around the age of six or seven.

Also, there are a substantial number of children with either congenital amputations or with amputations resulting from accidents who are treated by pediatric orthopedists for the fitting of prostheses (artificial limbs).

Some of the outstanding pediatric orthopedic surgeons on this list also perform adult orthopedic surgery.

PEDIATRIC ORTHOPEDIC SURGEONS

Dr. David S. Bradford
University of Minnesota Hospitals
Minneapolis, Minnesota 55455

Professor of orthopedics.

Dr. Wilton Bunch
Loyola University Medical School
Maywood, Illinois 60153

Professor of orthopedic surgery.

Dr. Sherman S. Coleman
University of Utah Medical Center
Salt Lake City, Utah 84132

Professor of surgery.

Dr. Albert B. Ferguson, Jr.
Children's Hospital
Pittsburgh, Pennsylvania 15213

David Silver professor of orthopedic surgery, University of Pittsburgh Medical School.

Dr. Paul P. Griffin
Vanderbilt University
Medical Center
Nashville, Tennessee 37203

Professor and chairman, department of orthopedics.

Dr. John E. Hall
Children's Hospital
300 Longwood Avenue
Boston, Massachusetts 02115

Professor of orthopedic surgery, Harvard; chief of clinical orthopedics, Children's Hospital. Known for his work with scoliosis.

Dr. Wood W. Lovell
1001 Johnson Ferry Road, NE
Atlanta, Georgia 30342

Medical director and pediatric orthopedic surgeon, Scottish Rite Hospital.

Dr. Dean G. MacEwen
Alfred I. Du Pont Institute
Wilmington, Delaware 19899

Medical director, Alfred I. Du Pont Institute; professor of orthopedic surgery, Jefferson Medical College in Philadelphia.

Dr. Douglas W. McKay
Children's Hospital National
Medical Center
111 Michigan Avenue, NW
Washington, District of Columbia
20010

Surgeon-in-chief.

Dr. Robert Siffert
Mt. Sinai Hospital
New York, New York 10029

Professor and chairman, department of orthopedic surgery.

Dr. Lynn T. Staheli
Children's Orthopedic Hospital
4800 Sand Point Way, NE
Seattle, Washington 98105

Clinical associate professor of orthopedics, University of Washington.

Dr. Howard Steel
Shriner's Hospital for Crippled
Children
Philadelphia, Pennsylvania 19152

Chief surgeon at Shriner's and Children's Hospital; professor of orthopedic surgery, Temple University.

Dr. Frank H. Stelling
Piedmont Orthopedic Clinic
1050 Grove Road
Greenville, South Carolina 29605

Chief surgeon, Shriner's Hospital.

Dr. Mihran O. Tachdjian
Children's Memorial Hospital
Chicago, Illinois 60614

Professor of surgery, Northwestern Medical School.

Dr. G. Wilbur Weston
2300 South Hope Street
Los Angeles, California 90007

Clinical professor of surgery and orthopedics, University of California at Los Angeles Medical School.

Dr. John C. Wilson, Jr.
Children's Hospital
Los Angeles, California 90054

Chief of orthopedics; clinical professor of orthopedics, University of Southern California Medical School.

Dr. Robert B. Winter
Fairview–St. Mary's
Medical Building
606 24th Avenue South
Minneapolis, Minnesota 55454

Professor of orthopedic surgery, University of Minnesota. Known for his work on scoliosis.

Diseases of the Skin

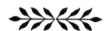

Pediatric Dermatologists

There are literally hundreds of skin diseases which can strike children. Many are inherited or congenital, and in a number of cases they require specialized treatment from a pediatric dermatologist. One pediatric dermatologist noted: "The average dermatologist does not know much about children and the average pediatrician does not know much about skin disease, so those of us who specialize in pediatric dermatology fill in this gap, especially in the treatment of the more complex or rare skin diseases of childhood."

As in all of pediatric medicine, the diseases that affect children must often be treated differently from the same diseases that strike adults. Some treatments for skin diseases that are fully acceptable for adult patients are totally inappropriate for a child. For example, a potent drug called methotrexate is sometimes used on adults in the treatment of disabling or severe psoriasis. However, if this drug were used on a child with psoriasis, according to one pediatric dermatologist, "it would be a disaster for that child." Thus, pediatric dermatologists are trained not only in the diagnosis and treatment of skin diseases, but in the growth and development of children and how this influences the disease and the treatment.

In addition to childhood psoriasis, pediatric dermatologists treat a wide range of skin diseases and disorders, including complicated acne, eczema, immunological disorders, unusual birthmarks, and a larger number of other, rarer skin problems. In cases of serious inherited skin disorders, an exact diagnosis is required in order to give the parents the full benefit of genetic counseling so they can be fully advised of the probability of any future child having the same disease.

Pediatric dermatology is not a separate, board-certified subspecialty. However, the dermatologists listed here are noted for their special expertise in childhood skin disorders. Most are trained and board certified in dermatology and pediatrics.

PEDIATRIC DERMATOLOGISTS

Dr. Nancy Esterly
Children's Memorial Hospital
Chicago, Illinois 60614

Professor of pediatrics and dermatology, Northwestern University.

Dr. Sidney Hurwitz
2 Church Street South
New Haven, Connecticut 06510

Associate clinical professor of dermatology and pediatrics, Yale University.

Dr. Alvin Jacobs
Stanford University Medical Center
Stanford, California 94305

Professor of pediatrics and dermatology.

Dr. Michael T. Jarratt
6655 Travis Street
Houston, Texas 77030

Associate professor of dermatology, Baylor College of Medicine.

Dr. Arthur L. Norins
University of Indiana
Medical Center
Indianapolis, Indiana 46202

Professor and chairman, department of dermatology.

Dr. James E. Rasmussen
University of Michigan
Medical Center
Ann Arbor, Michigan 48109

Associate professor of dermatology.

Dr. Lawrence M. Solomon
University of Illinois Medical Center
Chicago, Illinois 60612

Professor and chairman, department of dermatology.

Dr. Samuel Weinberg
2035 Lakeville Road
New Hyde Park, New York 11040

Associate professor of clinical dermatology and chief of pediatric dermatology, New York University.

Dr. William Weston
University of Colorado
Medical Center
Denver, Colorado 80220

Professor and chairman, department of dermatology.

Endocrine Disorders

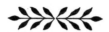

Pediatric Endocrinologists

Like adult endocrinologists, pediatric endocrinologists treat problems of the secreting glands. In particular, the endocrine glands include the thyroid, adrenal glands, pituitary gland, parathyroid glands, and reproductive glands, which all secrete hormones into the bloodstream, where they are carried to various cells and tissues to carry out their specific function. Lymph nodes, which often swell in the neck during infections and can be easily felt, are not in the province of endocrinologists because the lymph glands are not secreting glands. Lymph nodes catch germs and other poisonous substances in the body.

Also like adult endocrinologists, some pediatric endocrinologists tend to specialize in diabetes (which involves abnormalities of secretion of insulin in the pancreas), and they are listed in a separate diabetes section. Some pediatric endocrinologists are involved in both areas and are listed in both sections.

By far the most common cause for referral to a pediatric endocrinologist is for growth problems. The parents of young boys fear their child will be too short, while the parents of young girls fear their child will be too tall. One pediatric endocrinologist referred to growth problems as "body image disorders" that are painful but not fatal. Another pediatric endocrinologist suggests that body image disorders can in fact be fatal because the unhappiness a person feels over his or her size can lead to suicide. Parents of these children also suffer considerably.

The question is, when is tall "too tall" and when is short "too short" and what can be safely done about it?

There is a general rule for excessive height called the "rule of elevens," which suggests that if a girl's chronological age is less than eleven years and her skeletal age (the maturity of her bones) is also under eleven and her predicted mature height exceeds 5'11", then she may be a candidate for growth therapy. In many cases, young girls are brought in too late for therapy. Said one pediatric endocrinologist: "I am treating one young girl now who will be in excess of six feet tall if she is untreated. I am treating her with estrogens, which is the way excessive height is treated. I have explained to her and her parents the benefits and risks of the therapy and on balance the parents thought the risk of the estrogen therapy was outweighed by the benefit of preventing her from growing to an ungainly height."

One clinical study of estrogen treatment for growth retardation was conducted between the years 1959 and 1973 at the Royal Children's Hospital in Melbourne, Australia. Of the 168 young girls selected for treatment, 87 were finished with their treatment and they grew an average of 1.38 inches less than their projected height of 5'11.7". It should be noted that the projected height of children can be done accurately and simply using accurate measuring devices.

A study done at the Massachusetts General Hospital, also for fifteen years, found that young girls treated with estrogens averaged 2.4 inches below their projected height.

However, the potential side effects of such treatment are not fully known at this time. Estrogens (the same substance used in oral contraceptive pills) are known to cause venous problems with some women. Additionally, the risks of long-range problems such as breast or gynecologic cancer are not known at this time. Said one pediatric endocrinologist: "Quite frankly, it is too early to make the final judgment as to the total safety of this treatment. All the women we have followed up in our studies are doing fine, they are all perfectly normal. But our follow-up was not long-term because we haven't been doing this long enough yet."

Some studies have indicated that women treated with estrogen have produced children and have not suffered any fertility problems. Thus, any treatment for growth disorders requires a thoughtful scrutiny of all the alternatives, by doctor, parents, and child.

Much more common than complaints about excessive height are fears of being excessively short. What is too short? Generally, any child who falls below the minimum on growth charts is too short. However, endocrinologists are quick to point out that growth comes in spurts and that an accurate growth chart over a number of years should be kept by pediatricians in order to gain a more accurate prediction of the mature height of a young boy.

One endocrinologist offered a rule of thumb to determine shortness. At birth the average infant is twenty inches tall. A year later he will be one and a half times that, or thirty inches. In the second year, he should grow another five inches and after that an additional two and a half inches a year until puberty. Anything less than two inches a year, or any interruption of the growth rate, may be a sign of abnormal growth.

Although much can be done for shortness caused by growth hormone or thyroid hormone deficiencies, nothing can be done to overcome genetics. If the parents of a child are short, then the child will likely be short, and there is no treatment available to overcome this. The children who must be treated are those whose growing pattern is disturbed because of a hormonal problem, such as hypothyroidism or growth hormone problem. Sometimes the cause can be nutritional, or sometimes other physical causes such as kidney, heart, or pulmonary disorders can be present and can be detected, but hormone treatment will usually have no effect on these conditions.

There are other problems pediatric endocrinologists deal with. Delayed or very early puberty can be treated as well as problems of sexual differentiation for very young children. "At times the sex of the child can be difficult to determine," an endocrinologist remarked. "There can be uncertainty as to whether the child is an underdeveloped male or overdeveloped female. We can usually correct this."

The pediatric endocrinologists listed here treat the full range of children's endocrine problems.

PEDIATRIC ENDOCRINOLOGISTS

Dr. Robert Blizzard
University of Virginia
Medical Center
Charlottesville, Virginia 22901

Professor and chairman, department of pediatrics; a pioneer in treatment of growth disorders.

Dr. Alfred Bongiovanni
Catholic University of Puerto Rico
Ponce, Puerto Rico 00731

Dr. George W. Clayton
Baylor College of Medicine
Department of Pediatrics
Houston, Texas 77025

Dr. William W. Cleveland
University of Miami Medical School
Department of Pediatrics
Miami, Florida 33152

Professor and chairman, department of pediatrics.

Dr. John D. Crawford
Massachusetts General Hospital
Boston, Massachusetts 02114

Chief, pediatric endocrine metabolic service.

Dr. John F. Crigler, Jr.
Children's Hospital Medical Center
300 Longwood Avenue
Boston, Massachusetts 02115

Chief, endocrine division.

Dr. Angelo M. DiGeorge
St. Christopher's Hospital
for Children
2600 North Lawrence Street
Philadelphia, Pennsylvania 19133

Chief, endocrine and metabolic division.

Dr. Allan L. Drash
Children's Hospital of Pittsburgh
125 DeSoto Street
Pittsburgh, Pennsylvania 15213

Professor of pediatrics, University of Pittsburgh.

Dr. Delbert A. Fisher
Harbor General Hospital
1000 West Carson Street
Torrance, California 90509

Professor of pediatrics and medicine, University of California.

Dr. Douglas S. Frasier
Pediatric Pavilion
University of Southern California
at Los Angeles–Los Angeles
County Medical Center
1129 North State Street
Los Angeles, California 90033

Professor of pediatrics.

Dr. Orville Green
Children's Memorial Hospital
2300 Children's Plaza
Chicago, Illinois 60614

Professor of pediatrics, Northwestern.

Dr. Melvin Grumbach
University of California
Medical Center
San Francisco, California 94143

Chairman, department of pediatrics.

Dr. Stuart Handwerger
Duke Medical Center
Durham, North Carolina 27710

Associate professor of pediatrics; chief of pediatric endocrinology.

Dr. Alvin B. Hayles
Mayo Clinic
Rochester, Minnesota 55901

Professor of medicine and pediatrics, Mayo.

Dr. Wellington Hung
Children's Hospital–National
Medical Center
111 Michigan Avenue, NW
Washington, District of Columbia
20010

Dr. Ann Johanson
University of Virginia
Medical Center
Charlottesville, Virginia 22901

Professor of pediatrics.

Dr. Selma Kaplan
Department of Pediatrics
University of California
Medical Center
San Francisco, California 94143

*Director, department of
pediatric endocrinology.*

Dr. Solomon Kaplan
University of California at
Los Angeles Medical Center
Los Angeles, California 90024

Professor of pediatrics.

Dr. Robert Kelch
University of Michigan
Medical Center
Ann Arbor, Michigan 48104

Professor of pediatrics.

Dr. Maurice Kogut
The Children's Hospital
4650 Sunset Boulevard
Los Angeles, California 90027

*Professor of pediatrics,
University of Southern California.*

Dr. Fima Lifshitz
North Shore University Hospital
Manhasset, New York 11030

Head of pediatric endocrinology.

Dr. Margaret H. MacGillivray
Buffalo Children's Hospital
Division of Endocrinology
219 Bryant Street
Buffalo, New York 14222

Professor of pediatrics.

Dr. Claude Migeon
Pediatric Endocrine Clinic
The Johns Hopkins Hospital
Baltimore, Maryland 21205

Professor of pediatrics.

Dr. Maria New
Department of Pediatrics
New York Hospital–Cornell
Medical Center
525 East 68th Street
New York, New York 10021

*Chairwoman, department of
pediatrics, Cornell.*

Dr. Salvatore Raiti
National Pituitary Agency
210 West Fayette Street
Baltimore, Maryland 21201

*Associate professor, University of
Maryland Medical School; director,
National Pituitary Agency.*

Dr. Alan D. Rogol
University of Virginia
Medical Center
Charlottesville, Virginia 22901

Assistant professor of pediatrics.

Dr. Allen W. Root
The All Children's Hospital
801 Sixth Street South
St. Petersburg, Florida 33701

*Professor of pediatrics,
Southern Florida Medical School.*

Dr. Robert L. Rosenfield
University of Chicago Hospitals
950 East 59th Street
Chicago, Illinois 60637

Associate professor of pediatrics.

Dr. O. Peter Schumacher
Cleveland Clinic
Cleveland, Ohio 44106

Dr. Edna H. Sobel
Department of Pediatrics
Albert Einstein Medical School
1306 Morris Park Avenue
Bronx, New York 10461

Professor of pediatrics.

Dr. Juan Sotos
Children's Hospital
700 Children's Drive
Columbus, Ohio 43205

Chief of endocrinology.

Dr. Robert A. Ulstrom
Department of Pediatrics
University of Minnesota Hospital
Minneapolis, Minnesota 55455

Professor of pediatrics.

Dr. Judson Van Wyck
University of North Carolina
Medical School
Department of Pediatrics
Chapel Hill, North Carolina 27514

Chief, pediatric endocrinology clinic.

Dr. Virginia Weldon
St. Louis Children's Hospital
St. Louis, Missouri 63173

*Associate professor, Washington
University Medical School.*

Juvenile Diabetes Specialists

Although juvenile diabetes is much rarer than adult-onset diabetes, it is usually a more virulent and difficult disease to treat. Occasionally, the first symptom parents will see is a diabetic coma. However, in most cases continual thirst, excessive urination, and weight loss despite a big appetite signal the onset of the disease.

Diabetes is classified as an inherited disorder, although there are many cases of juvenile diabetes in children where there is no apparent family history of the disease. There are probably several factors at work. There is growing evidence that some cases of juvenile diabetes may have a viral origin. Thus, some children who acquire the disease may get it as a result of a viral infection, although the suspicion remains that the children inherited at least a tendency toward the disease. Simply because there has been no family history of the *symptoms* of diabetes does not mean that members of a family have not been carriers. In many instances, carriers of the disease never have symptoms and do not know they are carriers. In some cases, carriers of the diabetic trait in the family have died at a younger age from something unrelated to diabetes. Thus, they never lived long enough to have any diabetic symptoms, but the genetic tendency for the disease remained in the family. Thus the viral and genetic origins are probably not mutually exclusive.

Juvenile diabetes specialists contend that any person under the age of twenty who is dependent on insulin should be completely evaluated at a diabetic center if he has not been already. Most children's hospitals have diabetes units for this purpose. In some cases, adjustments in insulin levels or in the diet can aid that person substantially. (See introduction to adult diabetes specialists for examples of poor diabetes management.)

As noted in the introduction to adult diabetes specialists, the juvenile diabetes specialists listed here often treat and manage adult diabetics, but the reverse is not usually true. Adult diabetic specialists do not as a rule treat juvenile diabetics. Thus, except for those physicians who are designated as pediatricians or who are listed at children's hospitals, the specialists listed here also treat adult diabetics.

One further note. Some of the individuals on this list see patients on a consulting basis only. However, in some rare cases where the disease may be unusual, they provide comprehensive care for the patient. The consultants are generally full-time at major medical centers. Clinical professors and physicians in private practice generally offer ongoing diabetes management, as well as offering the full range of services to diabetic patients.

JUVENILE DIABETES SPECIALISTS

Dr. Lester Baker
Children's Hospital
Philadelphia, Pennsylvania 19146

Dr. Robert Bradley
Joslin Clinic
1 Joslin Place
Boston, Massachusetts 02215

Joslin Clinic is considered a leading diabetes clinic in the country. There are several outstanding juvenile diabetes specialists at Joslin, including Doctors M. Donna Younger, Stuart Brink, and Charles Graham. Also noted for adult diabetes.

Dr. Oscar Crofford
Diabetes Research and Training Center
Vanderbilt University School of Medicine
Nashville, Tennessee 37232

Both adult and pediatric. Special emphasis on emotional problems of adolescents with diabetes.

Dr. Dewitt Delawter
5500 Friendship Boulevard
Suite 803M
Chevy Chase, Maryland 20015

Clinical professor of medicine, Georgetown University Medical School.

Dr. Allen Drash
Children's Hospital of Pittsburgh
125 De Soto Street
Pittsburgh, Pennsylvania 15213
Professor of pediatrics, Pittsburgh.

Dr. Donnell Etzwiler
5000 West 39th Street
Minneapolis, Minnesota 55416
A pediatrician.

Dr. Fredda Ginsberg-Fellner
Mt. Sinai Medical School
11 East 100th Street
New York, New York 10029
Associate professor of pediatrics.

Dr. Richard Guthrie
2221 North Hillside
Wichita, Kansas 67219
Professor and chairman, department of pediatrics, Wichita State Branch of University of Kansas.

Dr. Ronald K. Kalkhoff
8700 West Wisconsin Avenue
Milwaukee, Wisconsin 53226
Professor of medicine, Medical College of Wisconsin.

Dr. Harvey C. Knowles, Jr.
University of Cincinnati
College of Medicine
231 Bethesda Avenue
Cincinnati, Ohio 45267
Professor of medicine.

Dr. George Clayton Kyle
University of Pennsylvania Hospital
3400 Spruce Street
Philadelphia, Pennsylvania 19104
Assistant professor of medicine.

Dr. Ralph C. Lawson
301 NW 12th Street
Oklahoma City, Oklahoma 73103
Clinical professor of medicine, Oklahoma University.

Dr. Alfred R. Lenzner
3834 Delaware Avenue
Kenmore, New York 14217
Assistant clinical professor of medicine, State University of New York (Buffalo).

Dr. John S. Llewellyn
510 Heyburn
Louisville, Kentucky 40202
Associate professor of medicine, University of Louisville.

Dr. James M. Moss
1707 Osage Street
Alexandria, Virginia 22302
Clinical professor of medicine, Georgetown University Medical School.

Dr. Henry Oppenheimer
St. Louis University Medical School
141 North Mervamec Avenue
St. Louis, Missouri 63105
Associate professor of clinical medicine.

Dr. Jerome R. Ryan
Tulane Medical School
1430 Tulane Avenue
New Orleans, Louisiana 70112
Professor of medicine.

Dr. William Schneider
1776 Vine Street.
Denver, Colorado 80206
Assistant clinical professor of medicine, University of Colorado.

Dr. Peter O. Schumacher
Diabetes Unit
Cleveland Clinic
9500 Euclid Avenue
Cleveland, Ohio 44106

Dr. E. Paul Sheridan
1776 Vine Street
Denver, Colorado 80206

Professor of clinical medicine,
University of Colorado
Medical School.

Dr. Joseph C. Shipp
University of Nebraska
College of Medicine
Omaha, Nebraska 68105

Professor and chairman, department
of medicine.

Dr. Charles R. Shuman
Temple University Hospital
3401 North Broad Street
Philadelphia, Pennsylvania 19140

Professor of medicine.

Dr. Thomas G. Skillman
Ohio State University
Hospital Clinic
456 Clinic Drive
Columbus, Ohio 43210

Kurtz professor of endocrinology.

Dr. John Stephens
Good Samaritan Hospital
Portland, Oregon 97210

Dr. Karl E. Sussman
University of Colorado
Medical School
4200 East Ninth Avenue
Denver, Colorado 80220

Professor of medicine.

Dr. Luther Travis
Department of Pediatrics
University of Texas Medical Branch
Galveston, Texas 77550

Professor of pediatrics.

Dr. Fred W. Whitehouse
2799 West Grand Boulevard
Detroit, Michigan 48238

Head, division of metabolic
disease, Henry Ford Hospital.

Kidney and
Urinary Disorders

Pediatric Kidney Disorders

End-stage kidney disease (kidney failure) is very rare among children; about 1.5 per million are afflicted with it. However, there are a number of other pediatric kidney disorders which are more common and which can cause partial kidney dysfunction.

Nephritis is an inflammation of the kidney which can cause partial or full dysfunction of the kidneys. Also, accidents which damage a kidney severely enough to require removal often require specialized care. In cases where one kidney is removed, the remaining one assumes the function of both. Kidney infections and developmental and congenital defects can also cause kidney disorders and are treated by pediatric nephrologists.

The kidney is a remarkable organ, in that it can be severely dysfunctional and continue to serve the body's needs. This is both a blessing and a curse because the kidney can be seriously malfunctioning without showing overt symptoms. One symptom of kidney dysfunction in children is a failure to grow properly. "If a child is not growing normally," one specialist said, "one thing the pediatrician should begin to suspect is kidney disease."

All of the outstanding kidney specialists listed here provide dialysis services. Dialysis is used when the kidneys fail to function at all. When this occurs, kidney transplantation is often attempted. Centers where this is done are listed under the pediatric kidney transplant section.

PEDIATRIC NEPHROLOGISTS

Dr. Billy Arant
University of Tennessee
Medical School
Memphis, Tennessee 38103

Associate professor of pediatrics.

Dr. Martin DeBeukeloer
Medical University of
South Carolina
College of Medicine
Charleston, South Carolina 29401

Dr. Chester Edleman
Dr. Ira Greifer
Dr. Adrian Spitzer
Albert Einstein Medical School
Bronx, New York 10461

Dr. Edleman is chairman of the department of pediatrics.

Dr. Richard Fine
Children's Hospital
Los Angeles, California 90054

Director of hemodialysis and transplantation.

Dr. Warren Grupe
Children's Hospital Medical Center
Boston, Massachusetts 02115

Dr. Alan B. Gruskin
St. Christopher's Hospital
2600 North Lawrence Street
Philadelphia, Pennsylvania 19133

Professor of pediatrics,
Temple University Medical School.

Dr. Malcolm A. Holliday
Children's Renal Center
University of California
Medical Center
400 Parnassus Avenue
San Francisco, California 94143

Professor of pediatrics.

Dr. John Lewy
Tulane University Medical School
New Orleans, Louisiana 70112

Professor of pediatrics.

Dr. Peter R. Lewy
Children's Memorial Hospital
Chicago, Illinois 60614

Head, division of nephrology.

Dr. William B. Lorentz, Jr.
Bowman-Gray Medical School
Winston-Salem, North Carolina 27103

Associate professor of pediatrics.

Dr. Paul McEnery
Children's Hospital
Cincinnati, Ohio 45229

Associate professor of pediatrics.

Dr. Stanley Mendoza
University Hospital
San Diego, California 92103

Chief of pediatric nephrology;
professor of pediatrics,
University of California.

Dr. Alfred Michael, Jr.
University of Minnesota Hospital
Minneapolis, Minnesota 55455

Professor of pediatrics.

Dr. George A. Richard
University of Florida
Medical School
Gainesville, Florida 32601

Professor of pediatrics.

Dr. Alan M. Robson
Children's Hospital
St. Louis, Missouri 63178

Dr. Norman Siegel
Yale University Medical School
New Haven, Connecticut 06510

Dr. Jose Strauss
University of Miami Medical School
Miami, Florida 33152

Professor of pediatrics.

Dr. Luther B. Travis
University of Texas Medical Branch
Galveston, Texas 77550

Professor of pediatrics.

Dr. Robert L. Vernier
University of Minnesota Hospital
Minneapolis, Minnesota 55455

Professor of pediatrics.

Dr. James E. Wenzl
Oklahoma Children's Hospital
Oklahoma City, Oklahoma 73190

*Professor of pediatrics; head,
nephrology section.*

Dr. Clark D. West
Children's Hospital
Cincinnati, Ohio 45229

Professor of pediatrics.

Pediatric Urologists

The basic difference between adult and pediatric urology is that
pediatric urologists operate on congenital defects while adult urologists
operate on acquired problems.

The number of full-time pediatric urologists is very small because
the number of congenital urologic problems is small relative to other
medical problems. "There are really only a handful of pediatric urologists in the country," one pediatric urologist said. "Generally, the
surgeons who have been doing pediatric urology are adult urologists
who did it part-time."

Pediatric urologists do not subspecialize in specific urinary surgical
procedures. However, one congenital malformation, *bladder exstrophy*,
involves a serious malformation of the bladder, and two pediatric
urologists are noted for their work in this area. They are so identified.

In addition, another congenital abnormality called *hypospadias* (a malformation of the urethra in males and females) is a specialty of a two-doctor team, one of whom is a urologist and the other a plastic surgeon. The plastic surgeon is also listed under plastic surgery, and his special interest in congenital genital malformations is noted there also.

All the urologists listed here are pediatric urologists only, or general urologists who spend at least half of their time on pediatric urology. Urology involves the kidneys, bladder, urinary tract, testes, and penis.

PEDIATRIC UROLOGISTS

Dr. Terry D. Allen
Southwestern Medical School
Dallas, Texas 75235

Associate professor, urology.

Dr. A. Barry Belman
Children's Hospital–National
Medical Center
111 Michigan Avenue, NW
Washington, District of Columbia
20010

Professor of urology and child health development, George Washington University Medical School; chairman, department of urology, Children's Hospital.

Dr. Victor A. Braren
Vanderbilt Medical Center
Nashville, Tennessee 37232

Dr. Arnold Colodny
Children's Hospital Medical Center
300 Longwood Avenue
Boston, Massachusetts 02115

General pediatric surgeon who does considerable urologic work.

Dr. Charles J. Devine, Jr.
(hypospadias)
Dr. Charles Horton
Hague Medical Center
400 West Brambleton Avenue
Norfolk, Virginia 23510

Dr. Devine is a urologist; Dr. Horton is a plastic surgeon. They are known internationally for their work in hypospadias. Dr. Devine is professor and chairman, department of urology, Eastern Virginia Medical School.

Dr. John W. Duckett
(bladder exstrophy)
Children's Hospital of Philadelphia
34th and Civic Center Boulevard
Philadelphia, Pennsylvania 19104

Dr. Richard M. Ehrlich
University of California at
Los Angeles Medical Center
Los Angeles, California 90024

Dr. Blackwell B. Evans
Tulane University Medical School
New Orleans, Louisiana 70112

Professor of pediatrics, Tulane.

Dr. Casey Firlit
Children's Memorial Hospital
2380 Children's Plaza
Chicago, Illinois 60614

Dr. Robert A. Garrett
University of Indiana
Medical Center
Indianapolis, Indiana 46200

Professor of urology.

Dr. James F. Glenn
Duke Medical Center
Durham, North Carolina 27710

Professor and chief of urology.

Dr. Edmond T. Gonzales
Texas Children's Hospital
Houston, Texas 77030

*Assistant professor of urology,
Baylor.*

Dr. Willard E. Goodwin
Division of Urology
University of California at
Los Angeles Medical Center
Los Angeles, California 90024

Professor of surgery.

Dr. Donald B. Halverstadt
Oklahoma University College of
Medicine
711 Stanton Young Boulevard
Oklahoma City, Oklahoma 73104

*Clinical professor of urology;
chief of pediatric urology,
Oklahoma Children's
Memorial Hospital.*

Dr. W. Hardy Hendren III
Massachusetts General Hospital
Boston, Massachusetts 02114

*Professor of surgery, Harvard;
director, division of pediatric
surgery, Massachusetts General.
Like Dr. Colodny, a pediatric
surgeon who does considerable
urologic work.*

Dr. Robert D. Jeffs
(bladder exstrophy)
The Johns Hopkins Hospital
Baltimore, Maryland 21205

Professor of urology.

Dr. George W. Kaplan
7920 Frost Street
Suite 401
San Diego, California 92123

Dr. Panoyotis Kelalis
Mayo Clinic
Rochester, Minnesota 55901

Professor of urology.

Dr. Lowell King
Children's Memorial Hospital
2300 Children's Plaza
Chicago, Illinois 60614

*Surgeon-in-chief, Children's
Hospital.*

Dr. George T. Klauber
Newington Children's Hospital
Newington, Connecticut 06111

Director of urology.

Dr. Stanley Jay Kogan
Albert Einstein Medical Center
Bronx, New York 10561

*Assistant professor of urology
and pediatrics.*

Dr. Selwyn B. Levitt
Albert Einstein Medical Center
Bronx, New York 10461

*Director, division of
pediatric urology.*

Dr. John H. McGovern
53 East 70th Street
New York, New York 10021

*Clinical professor of surgery
(urology), Cornell; director of
urology, Lenox Hill Hospital.*

Dr. Charles B. Manley
Children's Hospital
St. Louis, Missouri 63110

Director of pediatric urology.

Dr. David T. Mininberg
1249 Fifth Avenue
New York, New York 10029

*Associate professor of pediatrics
and urology, New York
Medical College.*

Dr. Alan D. Perlmutter
Children's Hospital of Michigan
Detroit, Michigan 48201

Director of urology.

Dr. Victor A. Politano
Jackson Memorial Hospital
Miami, Florida 33136

*Professor and chairman, department
of urology, Miami.*

Dr. Alan B. Retik
New England Medical Center
171 Harrison Avenue
Boston, Massachusetts 02111

Clinical professor of urology, Tufts.

Dr. John P. Smith
Children's Hospital
Columbus, Ohio 43205

Dr. Edward S. Tank, Jr.
University of Oregon Health
Sciences Center
Portland, Oregon 97201

Professor of urology.

Dr. R. Dixon Walker
University of Florida
Medical School
Gainesville, Florida 32611

Professor of urology.

Dr. R. Keith Waterhouse
450 Clarkson Avenue
Downstate Medical Center
Brooklyn, New York 11203

*Professor and head, department
of urology.*

Dr. Robert M. Weiss
Yale University Medical School
New Haven, Connecticut 06510

Professor of surgery.

Dr. John R. Woodard
Emory University Hospital
1365 Clifton Road, NE
Atlanta, Georgia 30322

Professor of urology.

Pediatric Kidney Transplant Specialists

The kidney transplant teams listed in the adult section also perform transplant operations on young people. With very young children under the age of eight, however, some of the problems require special experience provided by fewer centers.

The centers listed in this section are either exclusively involved with pediatric kidney transplants or have performed a substantial number of them and are among the most experienced pediatric kidney transplant centers in the country.

The number of young children who would benefit from kidney transplants is much smaller than adults because of the relative rarity of total kidney failure among young children. However, the same problems in adult transplantation apply to pediatric transplantation: that is, to balance the amount of immunosuppressant drugs against the body's tendency to get infections when those drugs are used to stop rejection. It is a delicate balance, requiring sophisticated medical knowledge and experience to know how to adapt therapy and handle the other problems which arise in children following transplantation. See the adult section for guidelines on what constitutes good transplant statistics for a center, as well as the legitimate questions that should be asked of a kidney specialist who recommends a certain center. The nephrologist *must* know the experience of the center, its survival rate for the children, and the success rate of the transplanted kidney. If he doesn't, then ask why he is recommending the center in the first place.

PEDIATRIC KIDNEY TRANSPLANT SPECIALISTS

Dr. Gerald Arbus
Hospital for Sick Children
Toronto, Ontario
Canada M5G 1X8

Dr. Arbus is a nephrologist who heads the pediatric transplantation team.

Dr. Richard Fine
Children's Hospital
Los Angeles, California 90054

Dr. Fine is a nephrologist who runs the kidney transplant program. This center is the most experienced pediatric kidney transplant center in the country.

Dr. Raphael Levey
Children's Hospital
Boston, Massachusetts 02115

Dr. Levey is a pediatric nephrologist.

Dr. Paul McEnery
Children's Hospital
Cincinnati, Ohio 45229

Dr. McEnery is a pediatric nephrologist.

Dr. John Najarian
University of Minnesota Hospital
Minneapolis, Minnesota 55455

Dr. Najarian is a surgeon in charge of the transplant program. Also listed in adult section. Dr. Michael Mauer is the pediatric nephrologist who heads pediatric kidney transplants.

Dr. Luther B. Travis
University of Texas Medical Branch
Galveston, Texas 77550

Dr. Travis is a pediatric nephrologist who heads the transplant team.

Diseases of the Eye

Strabismus

The most common serious eye disorder in children is strabismus, a muscle problem of the eyes which causes crossed eyes. The problem may be corrected in several ways—by exercise, special glasses, special eyedrops, or by surgery. Although children have this disorder in numbers far in excess of adults, some adults do have it, and the pediatric ophthalmologists on this list treat some adult patients. The specialists on this list are known for their work in strabismus. However, other, less common childhood eye problems, such as glaucoma or congenital cataracts, are usually handled by adult ophthalmologists who specialize in those areas. The following ophthalmologists are noted for their work with strabismus.

PEDIATRIC OPHTHALMOLOGISTS

Dr. Leonard Apt
Jules Stein Eye Institute
University of California at
Los Angeles School of Medicine
Los Angeles, California 90024

Professor of pediatrics; chief of pediatric ophthalmology.

Dr. John T. Flynn
Bascom-Palmer Eye Institute
University of Miami
Medical School
Miami, Florida 33136

Dr. Eugene Helverston
University of Indiana
Medical Center
Indianapolis, Indiana 46202

Dr. Arthur Jampolsky
Pacific Medical Center
2340 Clay Street
San Francisco, California 94115

Center director.

Dr. Philip Knapp
Columbia-Presbyterian
Medical Center
635 West 168th Street
New York, New York 10032

Professor of clinical ophthalmology.

Dr. Marshall M. Parks
3400 Massachusetts Avenue, NW
Washington, District of Columbia
20007

*Clinical professor of ophthalmology,
George Washington University
Medical School; senior staff
ophthalmologist, Children's
Hospital.*

Dr. Gunter von Noorden
Texas Children's Hospital
6621 Fannin Street
Houston, Texas 77030

*Professor of ophthalmology,
Baylor College of Medicine.*

Ear, Nose, and Throat Specialists

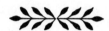

Problems Treated by Pediatric Otolaryngologists

Pediatric otolaryngologists perform most of their surgery to correct congenital defects of the ear, nose, and throat. Although some of them have special interests in certain aspects of ear, nose, and throat surgery, most of them perform the full range of surgery in this specialty.

Fluid in the ear is perhaps the most common problem children have that relates to this specialty, but there are other problems in which some pediatric otolaryngologists have a special interest. They are:

Endoscopy. This involves diagnosis of abnormalities and often the removal, by endoscope, of foreign matter from the larynx, lungs, or esophagus.

Stenosis of the larynx and esophagus. Stenosis, which means a narrowing or constricting, may be a congenital or acquired abnormality and can often be corrected by surgery.

Outer ear atresia. Atresia, which means the absence of, is another congenital condition which causes some children to be born without one or two ears. Surgical procedures have been devised to correct this condition.

Middle ear. Infections can cause damage to the eardrum. In some cases, surgery can repair it and restore at least partial hearing.

Deafness. Most causes of nerve deafness are irreversible, but in some cases deafness caused by anomalies can be restored, at least partially. One pediatric otolaryngologist listed here has as his special interest deafness in children.

A note of warning: Tonsillectomies are the procedures most frequently performed by ear, nose, and throat specialists and are, according to considerable evidence, one of the most overdone procedures in medicine. In 1975, in this country, 786,000 tonsillectomies were performed, a number some specialists find staggering. Many of these same specialists contend that many tonsillectomies could be avoided with little hazard to the child. The best specialists in this field only do tonsillectomies when there are clear and convincing indications for them.

PEDIATRIC EAR, NOSE, AND THROAT SPECIALISTS

Dr. Herbert Birck
Children's Hospital
Columbus, Ohio 43205

Chief, department of otolaryngology.

Dr. Charles Bluestone
Children's Hospital
Pittsburgh, Pennsylvania 15213

Director, department of otolaryngology. Known for middle ear work.

Dr. Francis I. Catlin
Texas Children's Hospital
Houston, Texas 77030

Professor of otolaryngology, Baylor College of Medicine. Noted for his interest in hearing preservation.

Dr. Seymore Cohen
1300 North Vermont Avenue
Los Angeles, California 90027

Clinical professor of otolaryngology and bronchoesophagology, University of Southern California. Known for his expertise with endoscopy.

Dr. Robin Cotton
Children's Hospital
Cincinnati, Ohio 45229

Director of pediatric otolaryngology; known for his work on stenosis of the larynx.

Dr. Blair Fearon
Hospital for Sick Children
Toronto, Ontario
Canada M5G 1X8

Noted for his interest in endoscopy.

Dr. Gerald Healy
Children's Hospital
Boston, Massachusetts 02115

*Otolaryngologist-in-chief at
Children's; associate professor
of otolaryngology at Harvard.*

Dr. Fred H. Linthecum, Jr.
Otological Medical Group
2122 West Third Street
Los Angeles, California 90057

*Clinical professor of otolaryngology.
Noted for ear work.*

Dr. David Mitchell
Hospital for Sick Children
Toronto, Ontario
Canada M5G 1X8

*Known for his work on outer
ear atresia.*

Dr. William Potsic
Children's Hospital
Philadelphia, Pennsylvania 19104

*Professor of otolaryngology,
University of Pennsylvania.*

Dr. Robert J. Ruben
Albert Einstein College of Medicine
Bronx, New York 10461

*Professor and chairman, department
of otolaryngology. A special
interest in deafness.*

Dr. Sylvan Stool
Children's Hospital
Pittsburgh, Pennsylvania 15213

*Professor of pediatrics and
otolaryngology, University of
Pittsburgh. Noted for his special
interest in endoscopy.*

Dr. Gabriel Tucker
Children's Memorial Hospital
Chicago, Illinois 60614

*Chief of otolaryngology; professor
of otolaryngology and maxillofacial
surgery, Northwestern University
Medical School. Noted for his
special interest in endoscopy.*

Allergies

Allergists and Immunologists

An allergy is a sensitivity to a substance to which most people have no reaction. The allergy may be to food, dust, pets, drugs, insect venom, or mold. An allergic reaction is a complex process, but as an example, take an allergy to pollen. In normal individuals, when the pollen is inhaled in normal breathing, pollen particles in the air are drawn into the nose, where they are deposited on the mucous membranes in the nasal passages. In normal individuals, the particles are moved through the nose by the cilia (the tiny hairs in the nose) to the throat, where they can be coughed out or swallowed.

However, in a person allergic to pollen, the process is different. The cells in the tissues under the mucous membranes are coated with a special kind of antibody, which, instead of helping that person fight off the inhalation of foreign particles, begins a harmful reaction which leads to the release of certain chemicals in the body. Once these chemicals are released, the person's allergic symptoms begin—whether it be sneezing, watery eyes, itching, or other symptoms.

Why some are allergic and others are not is uncertain. Heredity plays a role, but it is also clear that allergies cut across all lines of race, sex, and nationality.

Allergy and immunology are linked because allergic reactions are tied to a failure of the immune response in the body. Rather than creating an immunity, the antibodies do harm rather than good. Immunological problems are also part of other specialties, including dermatology (some dermatologists have special interests in immunological disorders of the skin) and rheumatology.

One of the most potentially dangerous allergic reactions is to insect bites, particularly bees, wasps, hornets, yellowjackets, and ants. Any one of these insects can, by one bite on an allergic individual, cause serious problems and, in some cases, death. In many cases there are warning signs. Most people who have a local reaction to a single sting often do not feel the need to consult an allergist. However, where a second sting causes a more severe reaction, experienced help should be sought. In some cases, in which the allergy to the insect is clear, allergy shots can be given to desensitize the individual to the insect's bites. While these shots do not work with every individual, many have reported an increased immunity to the insect bites after a full series of the shots. The newly available pure venoms appear to protect allergic people from the more severe reactions to insect stings.

Even if allergic reaction to the allergen cannot be prevented, skilled allergists have devised a series of precautions and therapies that help people live better with and avoid their allergies, whether it be asthma or insect bites.

Although *immunology* is not a separate specialty from allergy, some allergists have a special interest in immunological problems. Immunological problems in children (and adults) can cause an increased susceptibility to infections. Although many of the difficulties in combating immunological problems remain in the research stage, there have been some advances in recent years that offer some individuals an improved outlook.

The specialists listed below have special interests in allergy or immunology, or in some cases, they have special interests in specific allergies. When appropriate, they are so designated.

PEDIATRIC ALLERGY AND IMMUNOLOGY SPECIALISTS

Dr. D. C. Warren Bierman
(allergy)
University of Washington
Medical School
Seattle, Washington 98195

Clinical professor of pediatrics.

Dr. Rebecca H. Buckley
(immunology)
Duke University Medical Center
Durham, North Carolina 27710

Chief, division of allergy,
immunology, and pulmonary
disorders; associate professor
of immunology and pediatrics.

Dr. Elliot F. Ellis (allergy)
Children's Hospital
Buffalo, New York 14222

Professor of pediatrics,
State University of New York
at Buffalo.

Dr. Oscar L. Frick (allergy)
University of California
Medical Center
370 Parnassus Avenue
San Francisco, California 94122

Professor of pediatrics.

Dr. Elliot Middleton (allergy)
Children's Hospital
Buffalo, New York 14222

Professor of medicine and
pediatrics. A special interest
in asthma.

Dr. David S. Pearlman (allergy)
1450 South Havana Street
Denver, Colorado 80021

Clinical associate professor of
pediatrics, University of Colorado.

Dr. Frederick Rosen (immunology)
Children's Hospital
Boston, Massachusetts 02115

Professor of pediatrics;
chief of immunology.

Dr. Sheldon C. Siegel (allergy)
Allergy Medical Clinic
8540 South Sepulveda Boulevard
Los Angeles, California 90045

Clinical professor of pediatrics,
University of California at
Los Angeles; co-director,
pediatric allergy clinic.

Infectious Disease Specialists

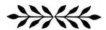

Experts in Infectious Disease and Their Special Interests

Like adult infectious disease specialists, pediatric infectious disease specialists always practice in hospitals, and most often university-affiliated hospitals.

They concentrate on diagnosing infections of undetermined origin, and then, when diagnosed, prescribe the proper treatment for the infection.

Another role they fill is to support the treatment of other diseases, most particularly, treatment of cancer and kidney disease. In treating these two diseases with immunosuppressant drugs, the body's resistance to infection is lowered significantly, and infectious disease specialists apply their skill to preventing and treating new infections.

Although pediatric infectious disease specialists practice the full range of diagnosis and treatment of infectious disease, many of them have special interests. These are:

Virus infections. Upper respiratory infections, some GI tract infections, as well as other types of infections are often viral in origin. In many cases, these types of infections can be very difficult to specifically identify. Unusual or complicated venereal diseases are treated by infectious disease specialists. Hepatitis, viral meningitis, and myocarditis also fall into this category.

Bacterial infections. Perhaps the most widely known and potentially one of the most severe of bacterial infections is meningitis. Also staphylococcal and streptococcal infections are bacterial. Infections of bones (osteomyelitis) and joints (pyogenic arthritis) are also bacterial.

Exotic infections. One specialist is noted for his interest in this area. One of the more well known infections in this group is smallpox. The last case in a natural setting occurred in October, 1977, in Somalia. There has been one laboratory infection in England since then.

Tropical diseases. Tropical or parasitic diseases, such as encephalitis, caused by viruses carried by insects, malaria, and worm infestations are a special interest of some infectious disease specialists.

Antibiotics. Although all infectious disease specialists have special interests in the use of antibiotics to fight infection, some have made this a special area of study.

Immune deficiencies. Those with a special interest in this area study how the body organizes itself to fight infection, and how that system fails in some people who seem especially prone to repeated infections. Specialists in allergy and immunology also study this area.

PEDIATRIC INFECTIOUS DISEASE SPECIALISTS

Dr. Charles A. Alford, Jr.
(infections in pregnancy and newborn infants)
University of Alabama
Birmingham, Alabama 35233

Professor of pediatrics.

Dr. Marc Beem (viral infections)
University of Chicago Hospitals
Chicago, Illinois 60637

Professor of pediatrics. Special interest in respiratory infections.

Dr. James Cherry (viral infections)
University of California at
Los Angeles Medical Center
Los Angeles, California 90024

Professor of pediatrics.

Dr. Floyd Denny (virus infections)
University of North Carolina
Medical School
Chapel Hill, North Carolina 27514

Professor and chairman, department of pediatrics. Has special interest in respiratory infections.

Dr. Heinz F. Eichenwald
(antibiotics)
Southwestern Medical School
Dallas, Texas 75235

Professor and chairman, department of pediatrics.

Dr. Ralph Feigin
(bacterial infections)
Baylor College of Medicine
Houston, Texas 77025

Professor and chairman, department of pediatrics.

Dr. Thomas Frothingham
(tropical diseases)
Duke University Medical Center
Durham, North Carolina 27710

Professor of pediatrics.

Dr. Lowell A. Glasgow
(viral infections)
University of Utah Medical Center
Salt Lake City, Utah 84132

*Professor and chairman, department
of pediatrics.*

Dr. Moses Grossman (antibiotics)
San Francisco General Hospital
San Francisco, California 94110

Professor of pediatrics.

Dr. Walter Hughes
(infections in cancer patients)
The Johns Hopkins Hospital
Baltimore, Maryland 21205

Professor of medicine.

Dr. Samuel Katz (central
nervous system infections)
Duke University Medical Center
Durham, North Carolina 27710

*Professor and chairman, department
of pediatrics. Special interests
also include viral infections.*

Dr. C. Henry Kempe (exotic
infections)
University of Colorado
Medical School
Denver, Colorado 80220

Professor of pediatrics.

Dr. Jerome O. Klein (antibiotics)
Boston City Hospital
818 Harrison Avenue
Boston, Massachusetts 02118

*Associate professor of pediatrics,
Boston University.*

Dr. Saul Krugman (viral infections)
New York University
Medical School
New York, New York 10016

*A special interest in hepatitis
(liver) infections. Professor of
pediatrics.*

Dr. I. George Miller
(viral infections)
Yale University Medical School
New Haven, Connecticut 06510

Associate professor of pediatrics.

Dr. Eric Ottessen (tropical diseases)
Building 5
Room 114
National Institutes of Health
Bethesda, Maryland 20014

*Parasitic diseases only. As with
all National Institutes of Health
care, it is free; but referrals are
required, and applicants must
fit within the National Institutes of
Health research protocols
established for their disorder.*

Dr. Robert Parrott (viral infections)
Children's Hospital National
Medical Center
111 Michigan Avenue, NW
Washington, District of Columbia
20010

*A special interest in viral
infections of the GI and
respiratory tract. Professor of
pediatrics.*

Dr. Stanley A. Plotkin
(viral infections)
Wistar Institute
36th and Spruce Streets
Philadelphia, Pennsylvania 19104

*Professor of pediatrics, University
of Pennsylvania.*

Dr. Paul G. Quie
(immune deficiencies)
University of Minnesota Hospital
Minneapolis, Minnesota 55455

Professor of pediatrics.

Dr. Arnold Smith
(bacterial infections)
University of Washington
Medical School
Seattle, Washington 98105

Associate professor of pediatrics.

Dr. Margaret H. D. Smith
(bacterial infections)
Ochsner Clinic
New Orleans, Louisiana 70121

*Professor of pediatrics, Tulane
University Medical School.*

Dr. Paul F. Wehrle
(bacterial infections)
C. D. Building
1200 North State Street
Los Angeles, California 90033

*A special interest in meningitis
and antibiotics. Professor of
pediatrics, University of Southern
California.*

Dr. Martha Yow
(bacterial infections)
Baylor College of Medicine
Houston, Texas 77025

Professor of pediatrics.

General Pediatric Surgeons

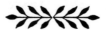

Areas Covered by General Pediatric Surgery

General pediatric surgery basically involves noncardiac surgery of the chest, surgery of the abdomen, and surgery of the head and neck, excluding orthopedic surgery and neurosurgery. Many general pediatric surgeons also perform urologic surgery, but because of the recent emergence of pediatric urology as a separate specialty, pediatric urologists are assuming more and more of the caseload in that area.

General pediatric surgeons perform the full range of surgical repair work necessitated by congenital abnormalities. The separation of Siamese twins and the repair of abdominal obstructions or malformations of the esophagus or trachea are some of the procedures which they perform. In the not-too-distant past, many of these congenital conditions resulted in early death or permanent disability, but they are now repaired successfully, allowing the child a normal life. Some pediatric surgeons also have a special interest in pediatric cancer surgery.

One particular operation for a congenital condition called *biliary atresia* has made substantial strides in the past few years. Formerly, biliary atresia*—a condition in which the bile flow from the liver to

* Atresia means absence; biliary refers to the bile duct.

the stomach is not possible because of the absence of the bile duct— was fatal in every case. However, recent strides have made it possible for more than a third of the children born with this condition to survive. Two pediatric surgeons are particularly noted for their work in this area.

Many of the pediatric surgeons listed here have special interests or particular expertise in various surgical procedures, but are not confined to these. When applicable, these special interests are noted. However, it should be emphasized again that all of the outstanding pediatric surgeons listed here perform virtually the full range of general pediatric surgical procedures.

GENERAL PEDIATRIC SURGEONS

Dr. Peter Altman (biliary atresia)
Children's Hospital–National
Medical Center
111 Michigan Avenue, NW
Washington, District of Columbia
20010

Professor of surgery, George Washington University Medical School.

Dr. William Clatworthy
(liver, tumors)
904 East Broad Street
Columbus, Ohio 43205

Professor of pediatric surgery, Ohio State.

Dr. Arnold Colodny
Children's Hospital Medical Center
Boston, Massachusetts 02115

Performs urologic surgery as well as general pediatric surgery.

Dr. Arnold G. Coran
C. S. Mott Children's Hospital
University of Michigan
Medical Center
Ann Arbor, Michigan 48109

Professor of surgery.

Dr. Alfred DeLormier
University of California
Medical Center
San Francisco, California 94143

Chief of pediatric surgery, Children's Hospital.

Dr. Angelo Eraklis
Children's Hospital
Medical Center
Boston, Massachusetts 02115

Associate clinical professor of pediatric surgery, Harvard.

Dr. Judah Folkman (cancer)
Children's Hospital Medical Center
Boston, Massachusetts 02115

Surgeon in chief; professor of surgery, Harvard.

Dr. Eric W. Fonkalsrude (chest)
University of California at
Los Angeles Medical Center
Los Angeles, California 90024

Professor and chief, department of pediatric surgery.

Dr. J. Alex Haller, Jr.
(chest, trauma)
Johns Hopkins Hospital
Baltimore, Maryland 21205

Professor of pediatric surgery.

Daniel Hays (cancer)
Children's Hospital
Los Angeles, California 90054

*Professor of surgery, University
of Southern California.*

Dr. Hardy W. Hendren III
Massachusetts General Hospital
Boston, Massachusetts 02114

*Known for urologic surgery, but
also performs general pediatric
surgery. Director of pediatric
surgery, Massachusetts General.*

Dr. Dale G. Johnson (trachea)
University of Utah Medical Center
Salt Lake City, Utah 84103

Head, division of pediatric surgery.

Dr. William B. Kiesewetter
Children's Hospital
Pittsburgh, Pennsylvania 15213

Professor of pediatric surgery.

Dr. C. Everett Koop (cancer)
Children's Hospital
Philadelphia, Pennsylvania 19104

*Professor of pediatric surgery,
University of Pennsylvania
Medical School.*

Dr. John Lilly (biliary atresia)
University of Colorado
Medical School
Denver, Colorado 80262

*Professor of surgery; chief of
pediatric surgery.*

Dr. Judson Randolph
(chest; esophagus; trauma)
Children's Hospital–National
Medical Center
111 Michigan Avenue, NW
Washington, District of Columbia
20010

Surgeon-in-chief.

Dr. Mark I. Rowe (newborn)
University of Miami Medical School
Miami, Florida 33152

*Chief, division of pediatric
surgery. A special interest in
metabolism of newborn children.*

Dr. Thomas Santulli (abdomen)
Columbia-Presbyterian
Medical Center
New York, New York 10032

Professor of surgery.

Dr. Samuel Schuster
Children's Hospital Medical Center
Boston, Massachusetts 02115

*Associate clinical professor
of pediatric surgery, Harvard.*

Dr. James L. Talbert (trachea)
University of Florida
Medical School
Gainesville, Florida 32610

Professor of surgery and pediatrics.

Dr. Morton Woolley
(chest; esophagus)
Children's Hospital
Los Angeles, California 90054

*Professor of surgery, University
of Southern California.*

Radiology

❧≫≫⟨⟨❧

Pediatric Radiologists

Although most laymen do not think of radiologists as specialists they can choose, radiologists think otherwise. There is considerable expertise in x-ray technique and interpretation. This is especially true in specialty areas and in pediatric radiology. "There are many diseases which are common to children which are not common to adults," one pediatric radiologist said, "and those experienced in pediatric radiology are more experienced in taking and reading x-rays of kids, and this gives us a distinct edge when the interpretation of the films is not obvious."

All children's hospitals have pediatric radiologists, and many major medical centers have specialists in pediatric radiology.

As noted in the adult section, if an x-ray is required, you are not bound to have it done at any one institution. You can have it done where you wish.

The physicians listed here are noted for their outstanding work in diagnostic pediatric radiology. Specialists in radiation oncology are listed in the cancer section.

PEDIATRIC RADIOLOGISTS

Dr. Ronald C. Ablow
Yale–New Haven Medical Center
789 Howard Avenue
New Haven, Connecticut 06504

Dr. Donald H. Altman
University of Miami Medical School
Miami, Florida 33152

*Clinical professor of pediatrics
and radiology.*

Dr. Walter Berdon
Columbia-Presbyterian
Medical Center
New York, New York 10032

Head of radiology, Babies Hospital.

Dr. Marie Capatanio
St. Christopher's Children's Hospital
Philadelphia, Pennsylvania 19133

*Director of radiology; professor of
radiology, Temple University.*

Dr. John Dorst
The Johns Hopkins Medical School
Baltimore, Maryland 21205

*Professor of radiology; associate
professor of pediatrics.*

Dr. Scott Dunbar
Children's Hospital
Cincinnati, Ohio 45229

Dr. Adele K. Friedman
Hospital of the University of
Pennsylvania
3400 Spruce Street
Philadelphia, Pennsylvania 19104

Associate professor of radiology.

Dr. Harold S. Goldman
Albert Einstein Medical School
Bronx, New York 10461

Professor of radiology.

Dr. Charles A. Gooding
University of California
Medical Center
San Francisco, California 94122

*Professor of radiology and
pediatrics.*

Dr. N. Thorne Griscom
Children's Hospital Medical Center
Boston, Massachusetts 02115

*Associate professor of radiology,
Harvard.*

Dr. Herman Grossman
Duke University Medical Center
Durham, North Carolina 27710

Professor of radiology.

Dr. John L. Gwinn
Children's Hospital
Los Angeles, California 90054

Radiologist-in-chief.

Dr. John A. Kirkpatrick, Jr.
The Children's Hospital
Medical Center
300 Longwood Avenue
Boston, Massachusetts 02115

Radiologist-in-chief.

Dr. Jerald P. Kuhn
Department of Radiology
Children's Hospital of Buffalo
Buffalo, New York 14222

Chairman, department of radiology.

Dr. William H. McAlister
Washington University
Medical School
St. Louis, Missouri 63110

Head of pediatric radiology.

Dr. William McSweeny
Children's Hospital National
Medical Center
111 Michigan Avenue, NW
Washington, District of Columbia
20010

*Director, department of radiology;
professor of pediatrics and
radiology, George Washington
University.*

Dr. William H. Northway
Stanford University Medical School
Stanford, California 94305

Professor of radiology.

Dr. Andrew K. Poznanski
C. S. Mott Children's Hospital
University of Michigan
Ann Arbor, Michigan 48104

Professor of radiology.

Dr. Bernard J. Reilly
Hospital for Sick Children
Toronto, Ontario
Canada M5G 1X8

Dr. Frederick Silverman
Department of Radiology
Stanford University Medical Center
Stanford, California 94305

Professor of radiology.

Dr. Edward B. Singleton
University of Texas at Houston
Houston, Texas 77030

*Clinical professor of diagnostic
radiology.*

Dr. Leonard Swischuk
University of Texas Medical Branch
Galveston, Texas 77550

Chief of pediatric radiology.

Dr. Hooshang Taybi
Children's Hospital Medical Center
Oakland, California 94609

Director, department of radiation.

PART IV

*Cancer and
Blood Diseases—
Pediatric and Adult*

Cancer Treatment—
A Blending of Specialties

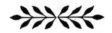

This special section is devoted to cancer because it is a disease that involves all parts of the body and all medical specialties. Because of the unique way the specialties are linked, coverage includes hematologists and oncologists who also treat *blood disorders* other than cancer.

Designed to be as comprehensive as possible regarding adult and pediatric cancer care, the following material includes:

1. *Pediatric and adult medical hematologists and oncologists.* These are specialists in chemotherapy who treat cancer and blood disorders.

2. *Adult and pediatric radiation therapists.* These are radiologists (also called radiation oncologists) who subspecialize in cancer radiation therapy.

3. *Gynecologic cancer surgeons.*

4. *Surgical oncologists.* These are most often general surgeons who have specialized in cancer surgery. This will include surgical specialists not found elsewhere, such as breast cancer surgeons.

5. *A key that indicates which medical and surgical specialties deal with certain types of cancer.* In each of the specialties, you will find some individual physicians who have special expertise in cancer.

6. *A listing of the 21 comprehensive cancer centers as designated by the National Cancer Institute.* Also included is a listing of cancer information numbers established by the National Cancer Institute.

These many different specialists are all included because cancer treatment usually requires a judicious blend of several specialties—

surgical, medical, and radiological. Because of the enormous complexity of cancer, and because no one can understand all aspects of it, there is an *absolute* need for multidisciplinary coordination in the effective treatment of cancer. At major medical centers, experts in diagnosis, oncology, cancer surgery, pathology, and x-ray therapy are available. These specialists often do cross consultation on cancer cases.

Although cancer remains the most dreaded disease in this country— a public opinion poll revealed that more Americans fear cancer than fear death—many significant strides have been made in recent years. Pediatric acute lymphatic leukemia is now responding extremely well to chemotherapy. Sixty percent of children with this disease have a five-year-or-more survival, and nearly 40 percent are cured completely with appropriate treatment. Treatment of Hodgkin's disease and related lymphomas has also resulted in significantly improved outlook for survival and cure. Sadly, in some cancers, such as lung cancer, there have not been significant strides in the past several years. However, by getting the best treatment, your odds of survival increase significantly.

One piece of advice every physician questioned gave was this: If you have cancer, go to a major medical center. Said one cancer specialist: "It is an extremely complex disease. No one person can treat it. A full team of individuals grounded in different approaches to the disease is required to get maximum benefit from cancer treatment."

Another piece of advice given by cancer specialists is that if you have cancer that requires surgery, be certain the surgeon you select has wide experience in cancer surgery. "It's not just the technical problem of removing the cancer," said one cancer surgeon, "it's understanding the biology of the disease and knowing when and where and how to operate on it that is important. You have to know how much tissue to remove or not to remove, and judgments such as this are best made by surgeons who operate on cancer often."

When one cancer specialist was asked what he would do if he had the disease, he said: "Putting myself in the place of a layman but with my knowledge, I would do this. If my family physician suspected I had cancer, I would ask for a referral to a medical oncologist or a medical specialist in the area of my cancer—such as a pulmonary specialist if I had lung cancer. I think too many people are not aware of this option. If you were told you had a heart problem, you wouldn't run off to see a heart surgeon; you would go to a cardiologist to evaluate your problem. I think a medical oncologist or specialist should serve the same purpose. He can serve as the patient's advocate.

"I think too often in the past when cancer was diagnosed, surgery was the only alternative. That is not always true today. Surgery may be indicated, but it may not be. I would trust my specialist to help me make those decisions and to assist in the treatment of my disease. There is no substitute for a *good* specialist in this disease."

There is a significant difference in adult and pediatric cancer, both in incidence, origin, and type of treatment. Thus, the specialist should be tailored to the age of the cancer patient. For example, in adults the common malignancies are known as carcinomas. In childhood, the cancers usually are sarcomas. Both are cancer, but they are different types of cancer, and the proper identification of the type and subtype of cancer is *crucial* in determining the appropriate therapy. This is another reason why a major medical center is vital for cancer care. The pathological examination of the cancer must be sophisticated and exact.

The difference between adult and pediatric cancer is perhaps most obvious in the types of cancers that strike these two age groups. In children, leukemia, central nervous system tumors (brain tumors mostly), and lymphomas account for more than 60 percent of all cancers. In adults, these three types of cancers account for less than 15 percent of all cancers. In children, lung cancer is virtually unheard of. In adults, it accounts for nearly a fourth of all cancers.

To reemphasize the most important advice cancer specialists gave:

1. Make certain you see a medical oncologist or specialist in the organ or system of your disease for evaluation for surgery *before* you see the surgeon.
2. If you need surgery, make certain the surgeon is widely experienced in cancer surgery.
3. Go to a major medical center or a specialized cancer center for treatment.

Hematology and Oncology

This section includes both adult and pediatric hematologists and oncologists. In pediatric hematology and oncology, the two specialties are linked as one. In other words, for a pediatrician to become a board-certified hematologist, he must pass the board qualifications for oncology as well. In adult hematology and oncology, this is not so, but the two specialties are linked because traditionally oncologists were also hematologists.

Thus, this section will include both specialties, but will indicate which hematologists and oncologists have a special interest in oncology, and which have a special interest in hematology. It should be emphasized, however, that the vast majority of hematologists and oncologists who appear in these lists are active in both hematology and oncology. In some cases, hematologists have special interests in certain blood disorders, and these are noted. Also, some have a special interest in certain types of cancer, and this is also noted.

The major special interests in pure hematology are:

Coagulation disorders. This includes many different disorders, but the major one is hemophilia. Major advances have been made in the treatment of this genetic blood disorder which allow hemophiliacs a better quality of life.

Anemia. There are several different types of anemia. Some are easily correctable with appropriate diagnosis and treatment; others are more persistent and virulent, such as *aplastic anemia*, which can be fatal.

Bone marrow transplantation. There are two centers in the country that have wide experience in bone marrow transplantation; they are nationally recognized. Both are listed under a special bone marrow transplant section. Bone marrow transplantation is still an experimental procedure performed for selected cases of aplastic anemia and leukemia. Although it represents a major advance in treating aplastic anemia, doctors warn that patients must not raise their hopes too high. Even in the best cases, only 50 to 60 percent of the patients appear to benefit significantly.

White cell disorders. The white blood cells are part of the body's immune, or anti-infection, system. When they malfunction, this can cause an individual to become susceptible to repeated infections. There is one pediatric hematologist and oncologist who has a special interest in this problem.

Hemoglobin disorders. The most widely known disorder in this category is *sickle cell anemia*, a blood disease which occurs in the black population. Some hematologists and oncologists—both pediatric and adult—have a special interest in this disorder.

Many of the specialists who have a special interest in oncology also have an additional interest in certain types of cancers, and these are so noted.

ADULT HEMATOLOGISTS AND ONCOLOGISTS

Dr. Raymond Alexanian (oncology)
M. D. Anderson Hospital and
Tumor Institute
Houston, Texas 77025

*Professor of medicine, University
of Texas Graduate School. A
special interest in myeloma.*

Dr. Daniel Bergsagel (oncology)
Ontario Cancer Institute
Princess Margaret Hospital
Toronto, Ontario
Canada M4X 1K9

*Professor of medicine at the
University of Toronto. A special
interest in myeloma.*

Dr. Joseph Bertino (oncology)
Yale University Medical School
New Haven, Connecticut 06510

*Professor of medicine. A special
interest in solid tumors.*

Dr. Clara Bloomfield (oncology)
University of Minnesota Hospitals
Minneapolis, Minnesota 55455

*Associate professor of medicine.
A special interest in leukemia
and lymphomas.*

Dr. George P. Canellos (oncology)
Sidney Farber Cancer Institute
Boston, Massachusetts 02115

*Associate professor of medicine.
A special interest in chronic
leukemia.*

Dr. Peter Cassileth (oncology)
University of Pennsylvania
Medical School
Philadelphia, Pennsylvania 19104

*Associate professor of medicine.
A special interest in leukemia.*

Dr. Samuel Charache (hematology)
The Johns Hopkins Hospital
Baltimore, Maryland 21205

*Professor of medicine. A special
interest in sickle cell anemia.*

Dr. Bayard Clarkson (oncology)
Memorial Sloan-Kettering Hospital
for Cancer and Allied Diseases
1275 York Avenue
New York, New York 10021

A special interest in acute leukemia.

Dr. Marcel E. Conrad, Jr.
(hematology)
University of Alabama
Medical Center
Birmingham, Alabama 35294

*Professor of medicine; director,
division of hematology and
oncology. A special interest in
anemia.*

Dr. Richard Cooper (oncology)
85 High Street
Buffalo, New York 14203

*Associate clinical professor of
medicine, State University of
New York. A special interest in
breast cancer.*

Dr. Jane F. Desforges
(hematology)
Tufts New England Medical Center
171 Harrison Avenue
Boston, Massachusetts 02111

Professor of medicine.

Dr. Vincent DeVita
Dr. Robert C. Young
Dr. Eli Gladstein
National Cancer Institute
Building 10
National Institutes of Health
Bethesda, Maryland 20014

Noted for ovarian carcinoma, lymphoma, and Hodgkin's disease treatment. Like all National Institutes of Health care, there is no charge. However, in order to be accepted for treatment you must be referred by a physician and you must meet the established National Institutes of Health research protocols. National Institutes of Health accepts most persons with Hodgkin's disease or lymphomas who have not had prior treatment.

Dr. John Durante (oncology)
University of Alabama
Medical Center
Birmingham, Alabama 35294

Director of the comprehensive cancer center.

Dr. Rose Ruth Ellison (oncology)
Columbia-Presbyterian
Medical Center
New York, New York 10032

Professor of medicine. A special interest in leukemia.

Dr. Clement A. Finch (hematology)
University of Washington
Medical School
Seattle, Washington 98105

Professor of medicine. A special interest in anemia.

Dr. Emil Frei III (oncology)
Sidney Farber Cancer Institute
Boston, Massachusetts 02115

Professor of medicine. A special interest in leukemia and lymphomas.

Dr. Emil J. Freireich (oncology)
M. D. Anderson Hospital and
Tumor Institute
Houston, Texas 77025

Professor of medicine, University of Texas. A special interest in leukemia and lymphomas.

Dr. Eugene P. Frenkel
(hematology)
Southwestern Medical School
Dallas, Texas 75235

Professor of internal medicine. A special interest in pernicious anemia.

Dr. William J. Harrington
(hematology)
University of Miami Medical School
Miami, Florida 33152

Professor and chairman, department of medicine. A special interest in immune disorders.

Dr. Robert C. Hartmann
(hematology)
University of South Florida
Tampa, Florida 33620

Professor of medicine. A special interest in anemia. Director of the section on hematology and oncology.

Dr. Paul Heller (hematology)
University of Illinois Medical School
820 South Damen Street
Chicago, Illinois 60612

Professor of medicine. A special interest in anemia.

Dr. Edward Henderson
(oncology)
666 Elm Street
Buffalo, New York 14263

Research professor of medicine, State University of New York. A special interest in leukemia.

Dr. James Holland (oncology)
Mt. Sinai Hospital
Fifth Avenue and 100th Street
New York, New York 10029

Professor and chairman, department of neoplastic disease. A special interest in leukemia.

Dr. Harry S. Jacob (hematology)
University of Minnesota Hospitals
Minneapolis, Minnesota 55455

Professor of medicine. A special interest in anemia.

Dr. Wallace N. Jensen (hematology)
Albany Medical College
Albany, New York 12208

Professor and chairman, department of medicine. A special interest in anemia.

Dr. Manuel E. Kaplan
(hematology)
University of Minnesota Hospitals
Minneapolis, Minnesota 55455

Professor of medicine. A special interest in anemia.

Dr. B. J. Kennedy (oncology)
University of Minnesota Hospitals
Minneapolis, Minnesota 55455

Masonic professor of medicine. A special interest in breast and testicular cancers and leukemia.

Dr. Burton Lee (oncology)
Memorial Sloan-Kettering
Hospital for Cancer and
Allied Diseases
1275 York Avenue
New York, New York 10021

A special interest in myeloma.

Dr. Lawrence S. Lessin
(hematology)
George Washington University
Hospital
Washington, District of Columbia
20037

Professor of medicine and pathology. A special interest in anemias.

Dr. Virgil Loeb, Jr. (oncology)
4989 Barnes Hospital Plaza
St. Louis, Missouri 63110

Associate professor of clinical medicine, Washington University. A special interest in leukemia and lymphomas.

Dr. Charles Mengel
(hematology)
University of Missouri
Medical Center
Columbia, Missouri 65210

A special interest in anemia.

Dr. Elliott Osserman (oncology)
701 West 168th Street
New York, New York 10032

Professor of medicine at Columbia University. A special interest in myeloma.

Dr. Saul A. Rosenberg (oncology)
Stanford University Medical Center
Stanford, California 94305

Professor of medicine and radiology. A special interest in lymphomas and Hodgkin's disease. Researchers at Stanford did much pioneering work in treatment of Hodgkin's disease and lymphomas, both in oncology and radiology.

Dr. Wendell Rosse (hematology)
Duke University Medical Center
Durham, North Carolina 27710

Chief of hematology. A special interest in immunological problems.

Dr. Wayne Rundles (oncology)
Duke University Medical Center
Durham, North Carolina 27710

Professor of medicine. A special interest in myeloma.

Dr. Sydney Salmon (oncology)
University of Arizona
Medical Center
Tucson, Arizona 85724

Director of the cancer center. A special interest in myeloma.

Dr. Philip Schein (oncology)
Vincent Lombardi Cancer Center
Georgetown University Hospital
Washington, District of Columbia 20007

A special interest in cancers of the digestive system.

Dr. John Ultman (oncology)
University of Chicago Hospitals
950 East 59th Street
Chicago, Illinois 60057

A special interest in Hodgkin's disease and lymphomas.

Dr. Ralph O. Wallerstein
(hematology)
3838 California Street
San Francisco, California 94118

Clinical professor of medicine, University of California. A special interest in anemias.

Dr. William J. William
(hematology)
State University of New York
at Syracuse
Syracuse, New York 13210

Professor of medicine. A special interest in coagulation problems.

PEDIATRIC HEMATOLOGISTS AND ONCOLOGISTS

Dr. Robert Baehner (hematology)
James W. Riley Hospital for
Children
Indianapolis, Indiana 46202

Professor of pediatrics and clinical pathology, University of Indiana. Special expertise in white cell problems.

Dr. James J. Corrigan, Jr.
(hematology)
University of Arizona Health
Sciences Center
Tucson, Arizona 85274

Professor of pediatrics. A special expertise in coagulation problems.

Dr. Audrey Evans (oncology)
Children's Hospital
Philadelphia, Pennsylvania 19107

Professor of pediatrics, University of Pennsylvania. A special interest in neuroblastoma.

Dr. Arnold I. Freeman (oncology)
Roswell Park Memorial Institute
Buffalo, New York 14263

Chief of the department of pediatrics. A special interest in acute leukemia.

Dr. John Hartmann (oncology)
Children's Orthopedic Hospital
and Medical Center
Seattle, Washington 98105

Chief of hematology and oncology.

Dr. George R. Honig (hematology)
Children's Memorial Hospital
Chicago, Illinois 60614

Professor of pediatrics, Northwestern University. A special interest in hemoglobin problems.

Dr. Norman Jaffe (oncology)
M. D. Anderson Hospital and
Tumor Institute
Houston, Texas 77025

A special interest in bone tumors.

Dr. Diane Komp (oncology)
Yale University Medical School
New Haven, Connecticut 06510

Professor of pediatrics.

Dr. William Krivit (oncology)
University of Minnesota Hospitals
Minneapolis, Minnesota 55455

Professor of pediatrics.

Dr. Sanford Leiken (oncology)
Children's Hospital–National
Medical Center
111 Michigan Avenue, NW
Washington, District of Columbia
20010

Chief of pediatric hematology and oncology.

Dr. Arthur S. Levine (oncology)
National Cancer Institute
National Institutes of Health
Bethesda, Maryland 20014

As in all National Institutes of Health patient care, there is no fee. However, patients must be referred and must meet the established National Institutes of Health research protocols for pediatric cancer. National Institutes of Health care involves many pediatric cancers.

Dr. Burton Lubin (hematology)
Children's Hospital Medical Center
Oakland, California 94609

Known especially for his expertise in sickle cell anemia and other hemoglobin problems.

Dr. Campbell W. McMillan
(hematology)
University of North Carolina
Medical School
Chapel Hill, North Carolina 27514

Professor of pediatrics. Known for his interest in coagulation disorders and in oncology, as well as for his interest in Wilm's tumor.

Dr. Alvin Maurer (oncology)
St. Jude Children's Research
Hospital
Memphis, Tennessee 38101

Medical director at St. Jude.

Dr. Howard Maurer (oncology)
Medical College of Virginia
Richmond, Virginia 23298

*Professor and chairman, department
of pediatrics. A special interest in
muscle tumors.*

Dr. Denis R. Miller (oncology)
New York Hospital–Cornell
Medical Center
525 East 68th Street
New York, New York 10021

*Professor of pediatrics; director
of pediatric hematology and
oncology at Sloan-Kettering
Hospital.*

Dr. Sharon Murphy (oncology)
St. Jude Children's Research
Hospital
Memphis, Tennessee 38101

*A special interest in non-Hodgkin's
lymphomas.*

Dr. David Nathan (hematology)
Children's Hospital Medical Center
Boston, Massachusetts 02115

*Professor of pediatrics,
Harvard. Known for special
interest in aplastic anemia.*

Dr. Thomas Necheles
(hematology)
New England Medical Center
Boston, Massachusetts 02111

*Professor of pediatrics at Tufts
University. A special interest in
aplastic anemia.*

Dr. Mark Nesbit (oncology)
University of Minnesota Hospitals
Minneapolis, Minnesota 55455

*Professor of pediatrics.
Known for his special interest
in acute leukemia.*

Dr. William A. Newton
(hematology)
Children's Hospital
Columbus, Ohio 43205

*Professor of pediatrics and
pathology. A special interest in
histological diagnosis.*

Dr. Frank Oski (hematology)
State University of New York
at Syracuse
Upstate Medical Center
Syracuse, New York 13210

*Professor and chairman, department
of pediatrics. Known for his
special interest in anemia.*

Dr. Howard A. Pearson
(hematology)
Yale University Medical School
New Haven, Connecticut 06510

*Professor and chairman, department
of pediatrics. Known for his
special interest in thalassemia.*

Dr. Gerald Rosen (oncology)
Sloan-Kettering Memorial
Hospital for Cancer and
Allied Diseases
1275 York Avenue
New York, New York 10021

*Associate professor of pediatrics
at Cornell University. A special
interest in bone tumors.*

Dr. Alan Schwartz (oncology)
University of Maryland
Baltimore, Maryland 21201

Associate professor of pediatrics.
A special interest in leukemia.

Dr. Stuart E. Siegel (oncology)
Children's Hospital
Los Angeles, California 90054

Head of hematology and oncology.
A special interest in neuroblastoma.

Dr. Lucius F. Sinks (oncology)
Lombardi Cancer Center
Georgetown University Hospital
Washington, District of Columbia
20007

Professor of pediatrics. A special
interest in brain tumors and
adolescents with cancer.

Dr. Margaret Sullivan (oncology)
M. D. Anderson Hospital and
Tumor Institute
Houston, Texas 77025

Dr. Charlotte Tan (oncology)
Sloan-Kettering Memorial
Hospital for Cancer and
Allied Diseases
1275 York Avenue
New York, New York 10021

A special interest in leukemia and
lymphomas.

Dr. John Truman (oncology)
Massachusetts General Hospital
Boston, Massachusetts 02114

Associate professor of pediatrics,
Harvard. A special interest in
leukemia.

Dr. Teresa Vietti (oncology)
St. Louis Children's Hospital
St. Louis, Missouri 63110

Professor of pediatrics,
Washington University. A
special interest in sarcomas
and leukemias.

Dr. Norma Sternberg Wollner
(oncology)
Sloan-Kettering Memorial
Hospital for Cancer and
Allied Diseases
1275 York Avenue
New York, New York 10021

Associate professor of pediatrics,
Cornell University. A special
interest in lymphomas.

Dr. William Zinkham
(hematology)
The Johns Hopkins Hospital
Baltimore, Maryland 21205

Professor of pediatrics.
A special interest in anemia.

Bone Marrow Transplant Centers

Bone marrow transplantation is an exacting, risky procedure. These two centers, which perform both adult and pediatric transplantation, are the most established in the country.

SPECIALISTS AT BONE MARROW TRANSPLANT CENTERS

Dr. George Santos, chief
Bone Marrow Transplant Service
The Johns Hopkins Hospital
Baltimore, Maryland 21205

Dr. E. Donnall Thomas, chief
Bone Marrow Transplant Service
University of Washington
Medical Center
Seattle, Washington 98104

ADULT RADIATION ONCOLOGISTS

Dr. Malcolm A. Bagshaw
Stanford University Medical Center
Stanford, California 93405

Director of radiation therapy.

Dr. Luther W. Brady
Hahnemann Medical College
230 North Broad Street
Philadelphia, Pennsylvania 19102

*Professor and chairman, department
of radiation oncology.*

Dr. Chu H. Chang
Columbia-Presbyterian
Medical Center
New York, New York 10032

Head of radiation oncology.

Dr. Gilbert Fletcher
M. D. Anderson Hospital and
Tumor Institute
Houston, Texas 77030

Head of radiation oncology.

Dr. Melvin L. Griem
University of Chicago Hospitals
950 East 59th Street
Chicago, Illinois 60637

Professor of radiology.

Dr. Samuel Hellman
Harvard Medical School
Boston, Massachusetts 02115

*Director, Joint Center
for Radiation Therapy.*

Dr. Henry S. Kaplan
Stanford University Medical Center
Stanford, California 94305

*Professor of radiology. Did pioneer
work in radiation treatment
for cancer.*

Dr. Simon Kramer
Thomas Jefferson Memorial
Hospital
Philadelphia, Pennsylvania 19107

*Chairman, department of
radiation therapy.*

Dr. Seymour Levitt
University of Minnesota Hospitals
Minneapolis, Minnesota 55455

*Professor and chairman, department
of therapeutic radiology.*

Dr. John G. Maier
Fairfax Hospital
Falls Church, Virginia 22046

Head of radiation oncology.

Dr. William Moss
University of Oregon Health
Sciences Center
Portland, Oregon 97201

*Professor and chairman, department
of radiology.*

Dr. Carlos A. Perez
Mallinckrodt Institute of Radiology
St. Louis, Missouri 63110

*Director, division of radiation
oncology. Professor of radiology
at Washington University.*

Dr. Ruheri Perez-Tamayo
Loyola University Hospital
Maywood, Illinois 60153

*Professor of radiology; director
of radiation therapy.*

Dr. Theodore L. Phillips
University of California
Medical Center
San Francisco, California 94143

Head of radiation oncology.

Dr. William E. Powers
The Harper Grace Hospital
Detroit, Michigan 48201

Head of radiation oncology.

Dr. W. D. Rider
Ontario Cancer Institute
Princess Margaret Hospital
Toronto, Ontario
Canada M4X 1K9

Dr. Philip Rubin
Strong Memorial Hospital
Rochester, New York 14642

*Chairman, department of radiation
oncology, University of Rochester.*

Dr. Glenn E. Sheline
University of California
Medical Center
San Francisco, California 94143

Professor of radiology.

Dr. Jerome Vaeth
St. Mary's Hospital and
Medical Center
2200 Hayes Street
San Francisco, California 94117

Chief of radiation oncology.

PEDIATRIC RADIATION ONCOLOGISTS

Dr. Robert Cassady
Joint Center for Radiation Therapy
Harvard Medical School
Boston, Massachusetts 02115

Head of pediatric x-ray therapy.

Dr. Giulio D'Angio
Children's Hospital
Philadelphia, Pennsylvania 19107

*Chief of radiology; professor of
radiology, University of
Pennsylvania. A special interest
in Wilm's tumor (kidney tumor).*

Dr. Sarah Donaldson
Stanford University Medical Center
Stanford, California 94305

Head of pediatric x-ray therapy.

Dr. Omar H. Hustu
St. Jude Children's Research
Hospital
Memphis, Tennessee 38101

Head of radiology.

Dr. Bertha Jereb
Memorial Sloan-Kettering
Cancer Center
1275 York Avenue
New York, New York 10021

Head of pediatric x-ray therapy.

Dr. R. Derek Jenkin
Princess Margaret Hospital
Toronto, Ontario
Canada M4X 1K9

Head of pediatric x-ray therapy.

Dr. Melvin Tefft
Rhode Island Hospital
Providence, Rhode Island 02902

*Professor of radiology,
Brown University.*

Surgical Oncologists—
Breast, Melanoma, and Other Cancers

There is a largely unresolved debate in medical circles as to who is best qualified to do cancer surgery—cancer surgery specialists or specialists in the part of the body where the cancer strikes.

At major medical centers this debate is not relevant because most cancer surgery is performed with both a specialist in the particular area of the body and a cancer surgeon present in the operating room. One understands the particular system or organ of the body better, the other the nature of the disease better.

The specialists listed here are outstanding surgical cancer specialists. Most of them perform general cancer surgery, which includes the breast, head and neck, digestive system, and melanoma. However, some of them are particularly interested in certain cancers, and they are so identified. In one case, the surgeon performs breast cancer surgery exclusively.

Many general surgeons and endocrine surgeons also perform breast cancer surgery, and some of those listed in the appropriate sections of this book perform it. Breast cancer surgery is not considered a difficult technical procedure, but any surgeon performing it should have wide experience in cancer surgery because his assessment of what type of procedure he should perform is vital.

In general, the radical mastectomy, which is the removal of the breast, lymph nodes, and muscle tissue from the chest wall, is performed less often than it once was. This is largely because accumulated evidence suggests that women who have less mutilating operations have similar survival times as those who have the full radical mastectomy.

One of the country's leading breast cancer experts said: "There is no evidence to indicate that radical mastectomy should still maintain a place in the therapeutic armamentarium of this disease. At present, we are evaluating the worth of segmental mastectomy, i.e., the removal of the tumor." Although this expert did not have any figures on how many radical mastectomies versus modified radicals are performed in this country, he guessed that the modified radical is the most frequently performed operation for breast cancer. However, he noted there are a "substantial" number of surgeons who still do the full radical as a matter of routine.

Another breast cancer surgeon urged that any patient facing the prospect of breast cancer surgery ask the surgeon what type of procedure he is planning. If he plans a full radical, ask him why and ask him if he ever performs any other types of procedure. If he does not, then you may wish to seek other advice. Also, as noted earlier, if you are diagnosed with breast cancer (or any cancer) you should consult with a medical oncologist before selecting a surgeon.

"The main thing to look for," a breast cancer surgeon said, "is flexibility. You must have a surgeon who adapts his surgery to the situation, not one who is wedded to one procedure and one procedure alone. You don't want too little surgery which will increase your chances of recurrence, and you don't want too much when it may well be unnecessary."

Still another cancer surgeon said: "The doctor who takes care of the breast cancer patient must have a full understanding of the biology of the disease, must know when to utilize other therapeutic modalities, and must be prepared to take care of the patient for as long as this patient lives. There must be a personal commitment."

Other surgical oncologists on this list have special interests in other cancers. *Melanoma,* which is a cancer that originates in skin pigments (often an unusual change in a mole is the first visible sign of this cancer), can be very virulent. As in breast cancer, surgical treatment of melanoma (not to be confused with myeloma, a leukemic-type bone cancer) requires a full understanding of the biology of the disease.

Another type of cancer in which one of the listed specialists has a special expertise is *sarcoma,* a soft-tissue cancer. One of the soft tissues commonly involved is the muscle.

As already noted, and as you will see in the guide to other cancer specialists, many doctors who specialize in certain organs or systems of the body have special interests in cancer.

SURGICAL ONCOLOGISTS

Dr. Harvey Baker
2222 NW Lovejoy Street
Portland, Oregon 97210
*Clinical professor of surgery,
University of Oregon.*

Dr. R. Robinson Baker
(breast surgery)
The Johns Hopkins Hospital
Baltimore, Maryland 21205
*Director of the breast clinic;
surgeon-in-charge, oncology.*

Dr. Benjamin F. Byrd, Jr.
(breast surgery)
Vanderbilt Medical Center
Nashville, Tennessee 37232
Clinical professor of surgery.

Dr. Blake Cady (breast surgery)
Lahey Clinic
605 Commonwealth Avenue
Boston, Massachusetts 02215

Dr. T. K. DasGupta (melanoma)
University of Illinois
Oncology Clinic
840 Southwood Street
Chicago, Illinois 60612
Head of surgical oncology.

Dr. Donald Ferguson
(breast surgery)
University of Chicago Hospitals
950 East 59th Street
Chicago, Illinois 60637
Professor of surgery.

Dr. Bernard Fisher (breast surgery)
University of Pittsburgh
Medical School
Pittsburgh, Pennsylvania 15261
*Professor of surgery. The director
of the National Cancer Institute's
study on breast cancer.*

Dr. William S. Fletcher
(breast surgery)
University of Oregon Health
Sciences Center
Portland, Oregon 97201
Professor of surgery.

Dr. Frederick M. Golomb
(melanoma)
910 Fifth Avenue
New York, New York 10021
*Professor of clinical surgery;
director of cancer immunotherapy,
New York University.*

Dr. Robert Hermann (breast;
GI cancer surgery)
Cleveland Clinic
Cleveland, Ohio 44106
Head of general surgery.

Dr. Alfred Ketcham
(general cancer surgery)
University of Miami Medical School
Miami, Florida 33152
Professor of surgical oncology.

Dr. Walter Lawrence
(general cancer surgery)
Medical College of Virginia
Richmond, Virginia 23298
*Professor of surgery; director
of the comprehensive cancer center.*

Dr. LaSalle Leffall, Jr.
(general cancer surgery)
Howard University Hospital
2041 Georgia Avenue, NW
Washington, District of Columbia
20060
*Professor and chairman, department
of surgery.*

Dr. Charles McBride
(melanoma; breast surgery)
M. D. Anderson Hospital and
Tumor Institute
Houston, Texas 77025

*Also known for breast cancer
surgery.*

Dr. Donald L. Morton
(melanoma; sarcoma)
University of California at Los
Angeles Medical Center
Los Angeles, California 90024

*Professor of surgery; chief,
division of oncology.*

Dr. Yosef Pilch (breast surgery)
Harbor General Hospital
Torrance, California 90509

*A special interest in immunotherapy
for breast cancer.*

Dr. Edward Scanlon
(breast surgery)
Evanston Hospital
2650 Ridge Avenue
Evanston, Illinois 60201

*Professor of surgery, Northwestern
University.*

Dr. Robert Schweitzer
3232 Elm Street
Oakland, California 94609

*Associate clinical professor of
surgery, University of California.*

Dr. John Stehlin, Jr. (melanoma)
777 St. Joseph Professional
Building
Houston, Texas 77002

*Director of the Stehlin Foundation
for Cancer Research. Dr. Stehlin is
also a pioneer in heat treatment
for cancer, a treatment which is
still in the experimental stage.*

Dr. Jerome Urban (breast surgery)
Memorial Sloan-Kettering
Hospital for Cancer and
Allied Diseases
1275 York Avenue
New York, New York 10021

*Director of the breast cancer
service. Unlike the other surgeons
on this list who do general
oncologic surgery, Dr. Urban
specializes in breast surgery
exclusively.*

Gynecological Cancer Specialists

Gynecological cancer is the second most common cancer among women, with approximately 70,000 new cases in 1978. However, gynecological cancer is also one of the most curable of all cancers if detected early. Some gynecological cancers have a 90 percent cure rate if detected early.

The gynecological cancer specialists listed here do little else except operate on and treat gynecological cancer. They are trained not only in the surgical care, but also in radiation and chemotherapy. One of the easiest and most reliable methods of testing for gynecological cancer is the Pap smear, which many gynecological cancer specialists recommend be done every six months. "If these tests are done regularly and frequently," one gynecological oncologist noted, "then if a test is positive we can be relatively certain that the cancer is recent and we improve immeasurably our ability to completely cure the disease."

A note of warning. Hysterectomies are performed on 647 out of every 100,000 women in this country, a figure many experienced gynecologists find enormously large. Many hysterectomies are done for sterilization when a simpler, less dangerous, and less expensive tubal sterilization might have been equally effective. Also, some hysterectomies are performed to prevent the possibility of future disease, a procedure thoughtful gynecologists find excessive. Be certain the indications for a proposed hysterectomy are sound. The better gynecological surgeons, of course, only perform hysterectomies when there are clear and convincing indications for them.

GYNECOLOGICAL CANCER SPECIALISTS

Dr. Hervy E. Avetette
Jackson Memorial Hospital
Miami, Florida 33136

Professor of obstetrics and gynecology, Miami University Medical School; director of gynecological oncology, Jackson Memorial Hospital.

Dr. Hugh R. K. Barber
Lenox Hill Hospital
New York, New York 10021

Director of obstetrics and gynecology.

Dr. Richard Boronow
University of Mississippi
Medical Center
Jackson, Mississippi 39216

Professor of obstetrics and gynecology.

Dr. William T. Creasman
Duke University Medical Center
Durham, North Carolina 27710

Director, division of gynecologic oncology.

Dr. Philip J. DiSaia
University of California
Irvine Medical Center
101 City Drive South
Orange, California 92668

Professor and chairman, department of obstetrics and gynecology.

Dr. Leo Dunn
Medical College of Virginia
Richmond, Virginia 23298

Chairman, department of obstetrics and gynecology.

Dr. Arthur Herbst
University of Chicago Hospitals
950 East 59th Street
Chicago, Illinois 60637

Chief of oncology service.

Dr. Conrad Julian
Vanderbilt Medical Center
Nashville, Tennessee 37232

Head of gynecologic oncology.

Dr. Leo D. Lagasse
University of California at Los
Angeles Medical Center
Los Angeles, California 90024

*Professor of obstetrics and
gynecology; director of
gynecological oncology services.*

Dr. George C. Lewis, Jr.
Division of Gynecologic Oncology
Jefferson Medical College
1025 Walnut Street
Philadelphia, Pennsylvania 19107

*Professor of obstetrics and
gynecology; director of
gynecologic oncology.*

Dr. John L. Lewis, Jr.
Sloan-Kettering Memorial Hospital
for Cancer and Allied Diseases
1275 York Avenue
New York, New York 10021

*Professor of obstetrics and
gynecology; chief of gynecological
services, Sloan-Kettering.*

Dr. John Mikuta
Hospital of the University of
Pennsylvania
Philadelphia, Pennsylvania 19104

*Director, gynecological oncology
division.*

Dr. George W. Morley
University of Michigan
Medical Center
Women's Hospital
Ann Arbor, Michigan 48109

*Professor of obstetrics and
gynecology.*

Dr. C. Paul Morrow
1240 North Mission Road
Los Angeles, California 90038

*Professor of obstetrics and
gynecology, University of Southern
California Medical School.*

Dr. James H. Nelson, Jr.
Massachusetts General Hospital
Boston, Massachusetts 02114

Professor of gynecology, Harvard.

Dr. Roy T. Parker
Duke University Medical Center
Durham, North Carolina 27710

*Chairman, department of obstetrics
and gynecology.*

Dr. Felix N. Rutledge
M. D. Anderson Hospital and
Tumor Institute
6723 Bertner Boulevard
Houston, Texas 77030

Chief of gynecology.

Dr. Julian P. Smith
Wayne State University
College of Medicine
Detroit, Michigan 48201

*Professor of obstetrics and
gynecology.*

Dr. Richard E. Symmonds
Mayo Clinic
200 First Street, SW
Rochester, Minnesota 55901

*Professor of gynecology,
University of Minnesota.*

Dr. J. Taylor Wharton
M. D. Anderson Hospital and
Tumor Institute
6723 Bertner Boulevard
Houston, Texas 77030

Associate professor of gynecology.

Dr. Paul B. Underwood, Jr.
80 Barre Street
Charleston, South Carolina 29401

*Director of gynecologic oncology,
Medical University of South
Carolina College of Medicine.*

Key to Other Cancer Specialists

In virtually every medical specialty, some individuals have developed a special interest or special expertise in cancer. They are so designated in each of the specialties listed in this book. This is a key which serves to help you find these other specialists who deal with specific types of cancer. In all major medical centers, of course, cancer patients are evaluated by a large number of medical consultants with special expertise in this disease.

Site of the Cancer	*Specialists Who Treat It*
Bladder	Urologists
Kidney	Urologists
Prostate	Urologists
Testicular	Urologists
Pancreas	GI Surgeons & Gastroenterologists
Stomach	GI Surgeons & Gastroenterologists
Liver & Biliary Tract	GI Surgeons & Gastroenterologists
Colon & Rectum	GI Surgeons, Colon & Rectal Surgeons, & Gastroenterologists
Lung	Thoracic Surgeons & Pulmonary Specialists
Brain & Nervous System	Neurosurgeons & Neurologists
Pituitary Gland	Neurosurgeons, Neurologists, & Endocrinologists

Thyroid Gland	Endocrine Surgeons, Endocrinologists, & Nuclear Medicine Specialists
Adrenal Gland	Endocrine Surgeons, Endocrinologists
Head & Neck (& Larynx)	Ear, Nose, & Throat Specialists
Mouth	Ear, Nose, & Throat Specialists
Ear	Ear, Nose, & Throat Specialists
Esophagus	Thoracic Surgeons, GI Surgeons, Gastroenterologists, & Pulmonary Specialists
Trachea	Thoracic Surgeons, GI Surgeons, Gastroenterologists, & Pulmonary Specialists
Skin (not melanoma)	Dermatologists
Bone Tumors	Orthopedic Surgeons
Eyelids & Eye Orbit	Ophthalmic-plastic Surgeons
Solid Tumors in Children	General Pediatric Surgeons
Leukemia, Lymphomas, & Other Cancers.	See Medical Oncologists, Radiation Therapists, & other listings in this section.

Comprehensive Cancer Centers

The National Cancer Institute (NCI) of the National Institutes of Health has designated twenty-one medical centers around the country as comprehensive cancer centers. The centers not only provide a full range of cancer treatment, but they also participate in ongoing clinical studies to discover what new therapies might be useful for cancer treatment.

In the questionnaire sent to the 500 physicians in researching this book, the question was asked of them: Do you think the comprehensive cancer centers provide patients with outstanding cancer treatment? The overwhelming majority (87 percent) replied yes. However, a number of dissenters as well as a number of those who supported the comprehensive centers made the point that many medical centers provide superb cancer treatment and many of them have cancer centers of their own.

The choice of a hospital for cancer treatment is obviously a question for you and your doctor. By all means, you should go to a major medical center, whether it be a comprehensive cancer center or another major medical center.

Telephone numbers of the centers are listed which can provide answers to many questions. Also, the NCI cancer information service telephone numbers are included. The 800 numbers are toll free for in-state calls. Finally, you can also call the NCI patient information number, (301) 496-6641, in Bethesda, Maryland.

THE TWENTY-ONE COMPREHENSIVE CANCER CENTERS

Cancer Center of Metropolitan
Detroit
Detroit, Michigan
(1–800) 462–9191
(313) 833–1977

Cancer Communications for
Metropolitan Washington
Vincent T. Lombardi Cancer
Research Center
Howard University Cancer Center
Washington, District of Columbia
(202) 232–2833

Colorado Regional Cancer Center
Denver, Colorado
(303) 333–1516

Columbia University Cancer
Center–Institute of Cancer
Research
New York, New York
(212) 694–4161

Comprehensive Cancer Center for
the State of Florida
Miami, Florida
(305) 547–6920

Duke Comprehensive
Cancer Center
Durham, North Carolina
(919) 286–2266

Fox Chase Cancer Center
Philadelphia, Pennsylvania
(215) 728–2700

Fred Hutchinson Cancer
Research Center
Seattle, Washington
(206) 284–7263

Illinois Cancer Council
Northwestern University Cancer
Center
University of Chicago
Cancer Research Center
Rush–Presbyterian–St.
Luke's Hospital
Chicago, Illinois
(312) 346–9813

The Johns Hopkins
Oncology Center
Baltimore, Maryland
(301) 955–3636

Los Angeles County–University of
Southern California Cancer Center
Los Angeles, California
(213) 226–2371

Massachusetts Cancer
Information Service
Sidney Farber Comprehensive
Cancer Center
Harvard University
Boston, Massachusetts
(617) 732-3000

M. D. Anderson Hospital and
Tumor Institute
Houston, Texas
(713) 792-3245

Memorial Sloan-Kettering
Cancer Center
Memorial Hospital for Cancer
and Allied Diseases
Sloan-Kettering Institute for
Cancer Research
New York, New York
(212) 794-7982

Minnesota Cancer Council
Mayo Comprehensive
Cancer Center
Rochester, Minnesota
(507) 282-2511

Ohio State University
Comprehensive Cancer Center
Columbus, Ohio
(614) 422-5022

Roswell Park Memorial Institute
Buffalo, New York
(716) 845-4400

University of Alabama
Comprehensive Cancer Center
Birmingham, Alabama
(205) 934-2651

University of California at Los
Angeles Comprehensive
Cancer Center
Los Angeles, California
(213) 825-5412

Wisconsin Clinical Cancer Center
University of Wisconsin
Madison, Wisconsin
(608) 263-6808

Yale University Comprehensive
Cancer Center
New Haven, Connecticut
(203) 436-3779

The Cancer Information Service (CIS)

Cancer Information Service (CIS) offices are now in operation to answer telephone inquiries about cancer from the general public, patients and their families, and health professionals. Persons calling the CIS reach information specialists. Information about cancer causes, prevention, detection, diagnosis, treatment, and rehabilitation is presented in layman's language. The CIS can also provide information about medical facilities in the area, possible sources of financial aid, and physician consultation services. These are the CIS telephone numbers. Many are toll free for residents in the regions they serve.

CANCER INFORMATION SERVICES

California (from Area Codes 213, 714, and 805):   1–800–252–9066

Colorado: 1–800–332–1850

Connecticut: 1–800–922–0824

Delaware: 800–523–3586

District of Columbia Metro Area: 202–232–2833

Florida: 1–800–432–5953

Hawaii: Oahu 536–0111
  Neighbor Islands—Ask operator for Enterprise 6702

Illinois: 800–972–0586

Kentucky: 800–432–9321

Maine: 1–800–225–7034

Maryland: 800–492–1444

Massachusetts: 1–800–952–7420

Minnesota: 1–800–582–5262

Montana: 1–800–525–0231

New Hampshire: 1–800–225–7034

New Jersey: 800–523–3586

New Mexico: 1–800–525–0231

New York State: 1–800–462–7255

New York City: 212–794–7982

North Carolina: 1–800–672–0943

Pennsylvania: 800–822–3963

Texas: 1–800–392–2040

Vermont: 1–800–225–7034

Washington State: 1–800–552–7212

Wisconsin: 1–800–362–8038

Wyoming: 1–800–525–0231

ALL OTHERS AREAS (except Alaska): 800–638–6694

PART V

Special Centers

Pain Clinics

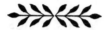

The overwhelming majority of people who come to pain clinics are addicted to prescription, pain-killing drugs. The director of one pain center reports that 85 percent of the patients who come to him for a consultation are addicted. The director of another pain clinic reports: "Our statistics indicate 94 percent of our patients are addicted, with Percodan (a frequently prescribed painkiller) the most common drug."

Besides addiction, there is one other significant statistic about people who come to pain clinics. They have had an average of *six* operations performed on them for relief of the pain.

Because of this, pain experts say that individuals suffering chronic pain should always do two things: Be wary of addiction to drugs, and do not have a surgical operation unless there is a very good diagnosis.

Pain clinics are a relatively new addition to medical care largely because pain has always been considered a symptom of a disorder, not a disorder in and of itself. This is still a sentiment that prevails throughout much of medicine. However, there are cases in which pain is both the symptom and the disorder, and must be treated. Thus, a new medical specialty, dolorology (from the Latin word meaning pain), has arisen.

Pain treatment centers use a variety of different techniques for ending pain. Nerve block techniques, biofeedback, electric current, hypnosis, and steroid injection are but a few of the techniques. The best pain treatment centers also involve a number of different specialists, including surgeons, neurologists, neurosurgeons, anesthesiologists, psychiatrists, and pharmacologists, who come together for the treatment and diagnosis of pain.

Back pain and headaches are by far the most frequent type of pain, but there are others as well. Phantom limb pain, in which great pain is experienced in a limb that has been amputated, is a frequent complaint. This psychosomatic problem requires considerable skill in treatment.

The following are the most established pain clinics in the country. When applicable, their special interest in certain kinds of pain is noted. Some are directed by neurologic surgeons, others by anesthesiologists, others by other specialists.

PAIN CLINICS

Dr. John Adams
Dr. Yoshio Hosobuchi
Pain Clinic
University of California Hospital
San Francisco, California 94122

Doctors Adams and Hosobuchi are co-directors.

Dr. Gerald Aronoff, director
Boston Pain Unit
Massachusetts Rehabilitation
Hospital
125 Nashua Street
Boston, Massachusetts 02144

Dr. John J. Bonica, director
Pain Clinic
University of Washington
Medical School
Seattle, Washington 98195

The oldest pain clinic in the country.

Dr. Verne Brechner, director
University of California at Los
Angeles Pain Management Clinic
University of California at Los
Angeles School of Medicine
Los Angeles, California 90024

*Specialists in nerve
block techniques.*

Dr. Steven F. Brena, director
Emory University Pain
Control Center
1441 Clifton Road, NE
Atlanta, Georgia 30322

Dr. David Bresler, director
University of California at Los
Angeles Pain Control Unit
405 Hilgard
Franz Hall
Los Angeles, California 90024

*Also a part of University of
California at Los Angeles, this
pain unit offers biofeedback,
relaxation techniques,
acupuncture, and others not
offered at the Pain Management
Clinic.*

Dr. Charles Burton
Dr. Charles Ray
Pain Clinic
Sister Kenny Institute
2545 Chicago Avenue
Minneapolis, Minnesota 55404

*Doctors Burton and Ray are
co-directors. Noted for back pain.*

Dr. Harold Carron, director
Pain Clinic
University of Virginia
Medical Center
Charlottesville, Virginia 22903

Dr. Benjamin Crue, director
Pain Center
City of Hope National
Medical Center
1500 East Duarte Road
Duarte, California 91010

Dr. Bertram Feinstein, co-director
Pain Center
Mt. Zion Hospital and
Medical Center
1600 Divisadero Street
San Francisco, California 94115

Dr. Edith Kepes
Dr. Norman Marcus
Pain Treatment Center
Montefiore Hospital and
Medical Center
Bronx, New York 10467

*Doctors Kepes and Marcus are
co-directors. Noted for treatment
of headaches.*

Dr. Donlin Long, director
Pain Treatment Center
Johns Hopkins University
Medical School
Baltimore, Maryland 21205

Dr. Ivan Podobrikas, director
Ohio Pain and Stress Center
1460 West Lane Avenue
Columbus, Ohio 43221

Dr. Max Sadove, director
Rush Pain Center
Rush–Presbyterian–St. Luke's
Medical Center
1725 West Harrison Street
Chicago, Illinois 60612

Dr. Joel Seres, director
Portland Pain Rehabilitation Center
Emanuel Hospital
3001 North Gantenbein Avenue
Portland, Oregon 97227

Dr. Frank Skultety
Dr. Bradley Berman, directors
Nebraska Pain Management Center
University of Nebraska
College of Medicine
42nd Street and Dewey Avenue
Omaha, Nebraska 68105

Dr. Richard Sternbach, director
Pain Treatment Center
Hospital of Scripps Clinic
La Jolla, California 92037

Dr. David W. Swanson, director
Pain Management Center
Mayo Clinic–St. Mary's Hospital
of Rochester
Rochester, Minnesota 55901
Inpatient pain center.

Dr. Josef K. Wang, director
Pain Clinic
Mayo Clinic
Rochester, Minnesota 55901
Outpatient pain clinic.

Dr. Alon P. Winnie
Pain Clinic
University of Illinois College of
Medicine
840 South Wood Street
Chicago, Illinois 60612

Sleep Disorder Centers

Virtually everyone at some time during his or her life suffers insomnia. In some cases, it can be persistent and aggravating. A number of well-controlled studies have proven beyond any doubt that sleeping pills have limited effectiveness—a very few days or weeks at most—and in many cases the pills can worsen sleeplessness. When insomnia is persistent and does not lend itself to the usual homemade methods we use to alleviate it—light exercise, relaxation techniques—a sleep center may offer help. Brain waves are monitored while you sleep—to determine how lightly or how deeply you sleep—and a number of other factors are studied. Also, other sleep problems, including restless leg, nightmares, night terrors, and a condition called sleep apnea, which causes some people to stop breathing temporarily while they sleep, can be treated.

Sleep researchers note that the best centers offer a full range of techniques and diagnostic methods to determine what is the source of the patient's sleeping problem—physical, emotional, or psychological. With an accurate diagnosis, the next step is to apply those treatment techniques which work best for the individual patient.

"Insomnia is a common problem," one sleep researcher said, "but its causes are unique to every person. There is no single solution to insomnia for everyone. That is one of the reasons sleeping pills fail. They are a blunt instrument where a very refined technique is needed. At the best centers, the patient's individual requirements are determined, and then treatment is expertly applied. This is why experience and expertise are so important."

There are no strict rules as to when your insomnia shifts from being a transitory problem to a serious one in need of expert attention. The judgment is the individual's and his family physician's. However, in the vast majority of cases if a patient tells his or her physician of a sleeping problem the answer is a prescription for sleeping pills. Although these pills have very limited usefulness in many cases, the prescriptions are filled and refilled for months and, in some cases, years. Said one sleep researcher: "One of the major problems we have with patients is that many of them are addicted to sleeping pills. They have to be withdrawn from the sleeping pills and then we can get to the basis of the sleeping problem. I think the evidence is clear and convincing that sleeping pills seriously exacerbate the problem of sleeplessness rather than improve it when taken regularly for an extended period of time."

What sleep researchers have also discovered is that people have very different sleep needs. Many people can exist on four or five hours a night, while some people need ten hours. "I remember one case of a woman who we studied who was in her late sixties and told us she had existed on one hour of sleep a night for as long as she could remember, back to her childhood. We tested her and found out two things. One is that she was right—she did only sleep one hour a night. But the most remarkable finding was that she had a very compressed sleep cycle. She went very quickly into the deepest and most restful stage of sleep and then came out of it quickly."

There are many sleep centers around the country. Those selected few listed here are the most established and have the greatest experience.

SLEEP DISORDER CENTERS

Dr. Roger Broughton
Ottawa General Hospital
43 Bruyere
Ottawa, Ontario
Canada K1N 5C8

Dr. Martin Cohn
Sleep Disorder Unit
Mt. Sinai Hospital
4300 Alton Road
Miami Beach, Florida 33141

Dr. William Dement
Stanford University Medical Center
Sleep Disorder Clinic
Stanford, California 94305

One of the preeminent sleep researchers in the world.

Dr. Peter Hauri, Ph.D.
Sleep Disorders Center
Dartmouth Medical Center
Hanover, New Hampshire 03755

Dr. Milton Kramer and
Thomas Roth, Ph.D.
University of Cincinnati
Sleep Disorder Center
Holmes Hospital
Cincinnati, Ohio 45220

Dr. David Kupfer
Western Psychiatric Institute
3811 O'Hara Street
Pittsburgh, Pennsylvania 15261

*Affiliated with the University of
Pittsburgh Medical School.*

Dr. Elliot D. Weitzman, director
Dr. Charles Pollak, co-director
Montefiore Hospital and
Medical Center
Sleep-Wake Disorder Unit
111 East 210th Street
Bronx, New York 10467

*One of the pioneer centers in sleep
research.*

Comprehensive Rehabilitation Centers—Pediatric and Adult

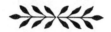

The rehabilitation centers listed here are noted for the wide range of expert rehabilitation services they offer. Rehabilitation from strokes is one of the most common reasons for rehabilitation centers, as is rehabilitation from arthritis.

However, there are a number of other accidents, illnesses, and birth defects which require rehabilitation and which these centers are equipped to handle. Spinal cord injuries, the aftereffects of cancer surgery, which can require a prosthetic device to replace an amputated leg or foot, brain injuries, cerebral palsy, and other birth defects all can require rehabilitation.

The best centers not only have an expert and experienced staff, but they have a staff large enough to perform the required rehabilitation work. "Rehabilitation is labor intensive," a rehabilitation expert said. "It requires a large staff to deal effectively with the problems our patients have. If the staff is insufficient, the patients suffer."

All of these centers offer many different rehabilitation techniques. There are also many smaller rehabilitation centers throughout the country which deal with individual problems, such as speech rehabilitation, arthritis rehabilitation, and other disorders.

COMPREHENSIVE REHABILITATION CENTERS—
PEDIATRIC AND ADULT

Dr. Arthur S. Abramson
Department of Physical Medicine
and Rehabilitation
Albert Einstein Medical College
1300 Morris Park Avenue
Bronx, New York 10461

*Professor and chairman, department
of physical medicine and
rehabilitation; director of the
rehabilitation center.*

Dr. Leonard Bender
Rehabilitation Institute of Detroit
261 Mack Street
Detroit, Michigan 48201

*Director of the center. Affiliated
with Wayne State University
Medical School.*

Dr. Henry B. Betts
Rehabilitation Institute of Chicago
345 East Superior
Chicago, Illinois 60611

*Professor and chairman,
department of rehabilitation
medicine, Northwestern University.*

Dr. Theodore Cole
Department of Rehabilitation
Medicine
University of Michigan
Medical Center
Ann Arbor, Michigan 48104

*Professor of physical medicine
and rehabilitation; director,
rehabilitation center.*

Dr. Paul Corcoran
Department of Rehabilitation
Medicine
University Hospital
750 Harrison Avenue
Boston, Massachusetts 02118

*Professor of rehabilitation
medicine; director, rehabilitation
center.*

Dr. Robin DeAndrade
Rehabilitation Research and
Training Center
Emory University
69 Butler Street
Atlanta, Georgia 30303

*Director, rehabilitation center;
professor of physical medicine.*

Dr. John A. Downey
Rehabilitation Medicine Service
Columbia-Presbyterian
Medical Center
New York, New York 10032

*Professor and chairman, department
of rehabilitation medicine.*

Dr. Jerome Gersten
Department of Rehabilitation
Medicine
University of Colorado
Medical Center
Denver, Colorado 80262

*Professor and head, department of
physical medicine and rehabilitation.*

Dr. Dorothea D. Glass
Moss Rehabilitation Hospital
12th and Tabor Roads
Philadelphia, Pennsylvania 19141

*Professor of rehabilitation medicine,
Temple University. Center known
especially for work in sexual
rehabilitation for arthritics.*

Dr. Ernest W. Johnson
Department of Physical Medicine
University Hospital
410 West Tenth Avenue
Columbus, Ohio 43210

*Professor and chairman, department
of physical medicine.*

Dr. Frederic J. Kottke
University of Minnesota
Rehabilitation Center
Minneapolis, Minnesota 55455

*Head, department of physical
medicine and rehabilitation.*

Dr. Justus F. Lehmann
Department of Rehabilitation
Medicine
University of Washington
Medical Center
Seattle, Washington 98105

*Professor and chairman, department
of rehabilitation medicine.*

Dr. Howard Rusk
Dr. Joseph Goodgold
Dr. Edward Lowman
Rusk Rehabilitation Institute
400 East 34th Street
New York, New York 10016

*All three are on the teaching faculty
at New York University Medical
School, with which the
Rehabilitation Institute is
affiliated.*

Dr. William Spencer
Texas Institute of Rehabilitation
Texas Medical Center
Houston, Texas 77025

Director of the center.

Dr. Samuel L. Stover
Spain Rehabilitation Center
University of Alabama
Medical Center
Birmingham, Alabama 35294

*Professor of physical medicine;
head, rehabilitation center.*

Dr. Robert Swezey
Arthritis and Back Pain Center
2200 Santa Monica Boulevard
Santa Monica, California 90404

*Director of the center. Noted
especially for arthritis rehabilitation,
back pain, and related disorders.*

Burn Centers—
Adult and Pediatric

In burn cases, as in all medical emergencies, the patient is usually taken to the nearest available hospital. However, in complex burn cases, such as burns of the hands or feet, or burns of the face, or third-degree burns which cover more than 15 percent of the body, a major burn center is usually recommended. Also, any burns from an electrical shock often require specialized care.

One burn specialist said the many major burn centers also take in people with relatively minor burns, so a serious burn is not a prerequisite for admittance. "If you are burned rather seriously," he suggested, "and you are taken to a local hospital, you should ask them very directly at that hospital if they have substantial experience with serious burn cases and if they think you should go to a major burn center. In most cases, if they think they can't handle it, they will agree to transfer you."

After initial shock, the major threat of serious burns is from infection, a threat which lasts throughout the healing process. Also, serious burns affect virtually every major system of the body as they react to cope with the injury. Many of the outstanding centers listed offer both adult and pediatric burn care; some offer only one. The Shriner's burn units around the country offer only pediatric care.

BURN CENTERS

Dr. Charles R. Baxter, chief
(adult and pediatric)
Burn Unit
Parkland Memorial Hospital
Dallas, Texas 75235

Dr. John F. Burke, chief (adult)
Burn Unit
Massachusetts General Hospital
Boston, Massachusetts 02114

Dr. John F. Burke, chief
(pediatric)
Burn Unit
Shriner's Hospital for Crippled
Children
Boston, Massachusetts 02114

Dr. P. William Curreri, chief
(adult and pediatric)
Burn Center
New York Hospital–Cornell
Medical Center
New York, New York 10021

Dr. B. W. Haynes, Jr.
(pediatric and adult)
Burn Unit
Medical College of
Virginia Hospitals
Richmond, Virginia 23298

Dr. David M. Heimbach, chief
(adult and pediatric)
Burn Center
Harborview Medical Center
Seattle, Washington 98104

Dr. Robert P. Hummel, chief (adult)
Burn Unit
Cincinnati General Hospital
Cincinnati, Ohio 45267

Dr. Bruce G. McMillan, chief
(pediatric)
Burn Unit
Shriner's Hospital for
Crippled Children
Cincinnati, Ohio 45219

Dr. William Monafo, chief
(pediatric and adult)
Burn Unit
St. John's Mercy Hospital
St. Louis, Missouri 63141

Dr. Donald Parks, chief
(pediatric)
Shriner's Burn Institute
University of Texas Medical Branch
Hospitals
Galveston, Texas 77550

*There is also an adult burn unit
within the same medical center.*

Dr. Basil Pruitt, chief
(adult and pediatric)
Burn Center
Brooke Army Medical Center
San Antonio, Texas 78234

*Mostly for army personnel and
dependents, but some nonmilitary
connected civilians are admitted.*

Dr. Judson Randolph, chief
(pediatric)
Burn Unit
Children's Hospital–National
Medical Center
Washington, District of Columbia
20010

Dr. Bruce Zawacki, chief
(pediatric and adult)
Burn Unit
University of Southern California–
Los Angeles County Medical Center
Los Angeles, California 90033

Hospitals and Clinics

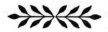

The questionnaire mailed to the 500 physicians as part of the research for this book included a question on their opinion of outstanding U.S. hospitals. Many responded by naming their own, others named hospitals with which they had been associated, still others named some which continue to have outstanding reputations in the medical community.

Although there was considerable disagreement about which hospitals were outstanding, there is little disagreement as to what the major ingredients are for a hospital to be outstanding. In short, those ingredients are the quality and depth of staff. One doctor said: "Some institutions become known because they have a few people with outstanding reputations. However, the best hospitals are those with depth in every department. I don't just mean a lot of people, but individuals with experience and specialized skills in every facet of medicine. To get this you need top-flight administrators at the top and in every department. If those administrators begin slipping, or a few key ones leave, a hospital can begin to suffer fairly quickly."

Most hospitals, even the most outstanding, usually do not have uniform depth and quality in every department. Some departments are more outstanding than others. Also, even in weaker hospitals, there may be departments which are more outstanding than those at the strongest hospitals. In selecting outstanding hospitals, the major criterion was across-the-board quality and strength.

Although there are many fine private hospitals in the country, those listed here are all university teaching hospitals, largely because they exist in a more self-critical environment than nonteaching hospitals.

While the quality of a hospital is vital, physicians who were interviewed on the subject insisted that the choice of doctor is usually more vital. The best doctors do not work out of inferior hospitals. And, even at the best hospitals, there are what one doctor called "two levels of care." He said one level was superior because the excellence of the physician demanded it from himself and from those attending his patient.

The hospitals and clinics included in this list are general care facilities. There are many, many smaller specialty care clinics throughout the country which often provide excellent care in a limited number of areas.

As a general rule, physicians said they believed larger hospitals offered significant advantages over smaller hospitals, and university hospitals were superior to nonteaching hospitals. Larger hospitals provide depth of staff in all of the major medical specialties which are crucial in diagnosing diseases as well as treating the more complex diseases. Teaching hospitals, they argue, offer a critical environment in which doctors are scrutinized and judged by their peers. They offered some general guidelines:

1. The hospital should have at least 400 beds.

2. Accreditation by the Joint Committee on Hospital Accreditation (JCHA) is a minimum requirement.

3. The hospital should be affiliated with a medical school.

4. Hospitals with American-educated interns and residents are greatly preferred over hospitals staffed by foreign-educated interns and residents.

HOSPITALS

Barnes Hospital
St. Louis, Missouri 63110

The medical faculty of Washington University practice and teach here.

Beth Israel Hospital
Boston, Massachusetts 02115

This hospital is part of the Harvard University system.

Columbia-Presbyterian Medical Center
New York, New York 10032

The major teaching hospital for Columbia University.

Duke Medical Center
Durham, North Carolina 27110

The major teaching hospital for Duke University.

The Johns Hopkins Hospital
Baltimore, Maryland 21205

The major teaching hospital for Johns Hopkins University.

Massachusetts General Hospital
Boston, Massachusetts 02114

The major teaching hospital in the Harvard University system.

New York Hospital–Cornell
University Medical Center
New York, New York 10016

The major teaching hospital for Cornell University.

Peter Bent Brigham Hospital
Boston, Massachusetts 02115

A small hospital, part of the Harvard University system.

Stanford University Medical Center
Stanford, California 94305

The major teaching facility for Stanford University.

Strong Memorial Hospital
Rochester, New York 14642

The major teaching hospital for the University of Rochester.

University of California at Los
Angeles Medical Center
Los Angeles, California 90024

The major teaching facility for the University of California at Los Angeles Medical School.

University of California
Medical Center
San Francisco, California 94143

The major teaching facility for the University of California.

University of Chicago Hospitals
Chicago, Illinois 60637

The major teaching facility for the University of Chicago.

University of Michigan
Medical Center
Ann Arbor, Michigan 48104

The major teaching facility for the University of Michigan.

University of Minnesota Hospitals
Minneapolis, Minnesota 55455

The major teaching facility for the University of Minnesota.

Yale–New Haven Hospital
New Haven, Connecticut 06510

The major teaching hospital for Yale.

CLINICS

The Cleveland Clinic
Cleveland, Ohio 44106

A private institution.

The Emory University Clinic
Atlanta, Georgia 30303

Affiliated with Emory University Medical School.

The Lahey Clinic
Boston, Massachusetts 02215

Largely a private clinic.
Some members of the Lahey staff
hold teaching positions at Harvard.

The Mayo Clinic
Rochester, Minnesota 55901

A private clinic which in
recent years developed its
own graduate school of medicine.

The Ochsner Clinic
New Orleans, Louisiana 70121

A private clinic.

NOTES

NOTES

NOTES

NOTES

NOTES

NOTES

NOTES

NOTES